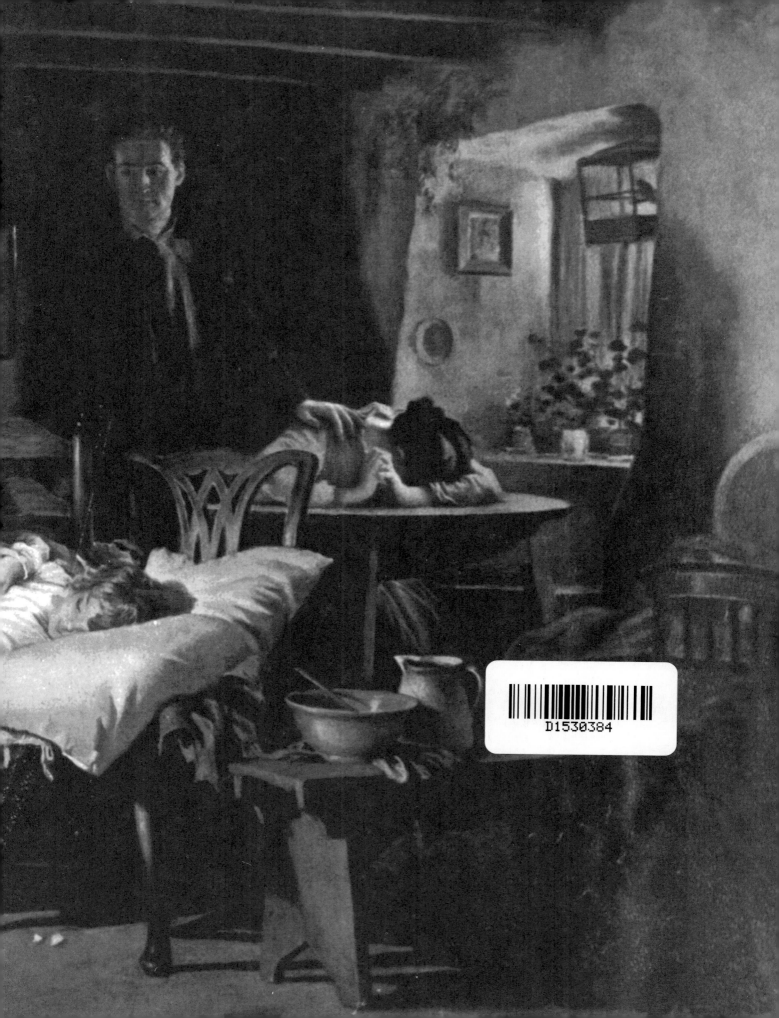

The American Academy of Family Physicians
is pleased to present

CARING FOR AMERICA
The Story
of Family Practice

by
John R. Stanard

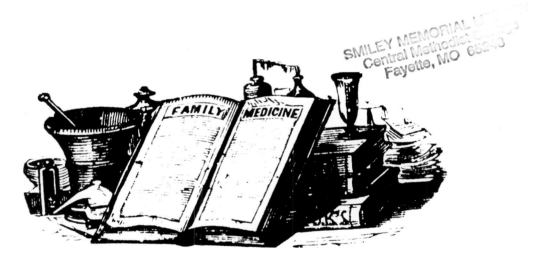

Illustration from Handbook of Early American Art
(State Historical Society of Missouri, Columbia.)

Proceeds from sale of this book will benefit the charitable endeavors of the
American Academy of Family Physicians Foundation.

This book is funded in part by a grant from Glaxo Wellcome Inc.

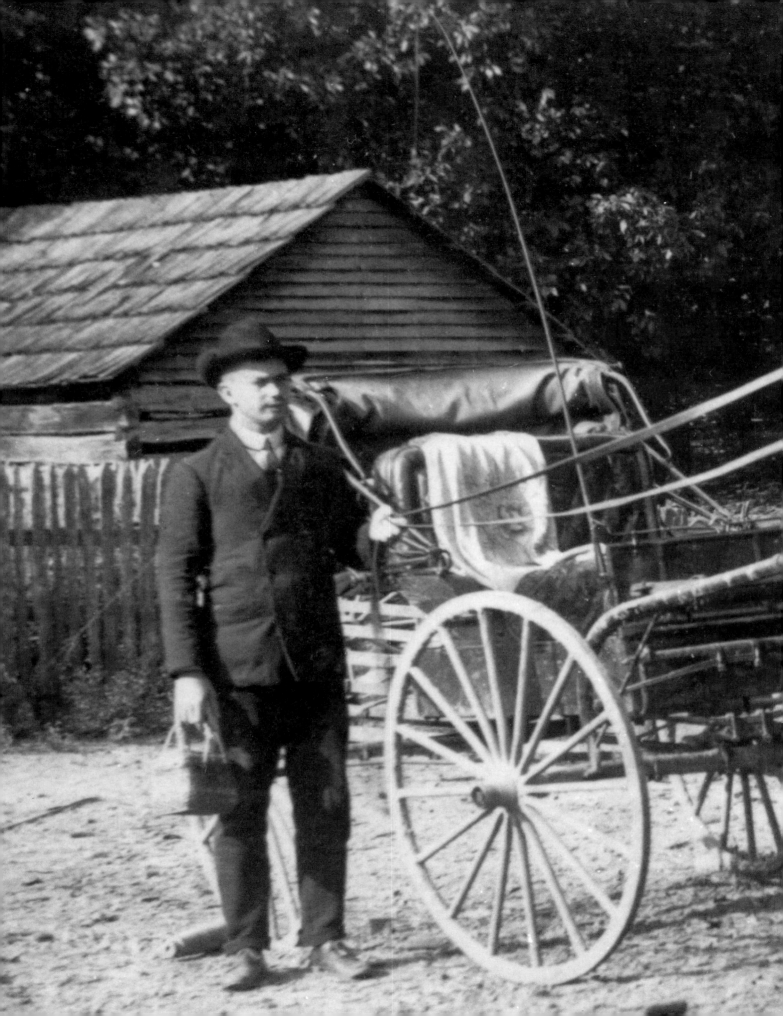

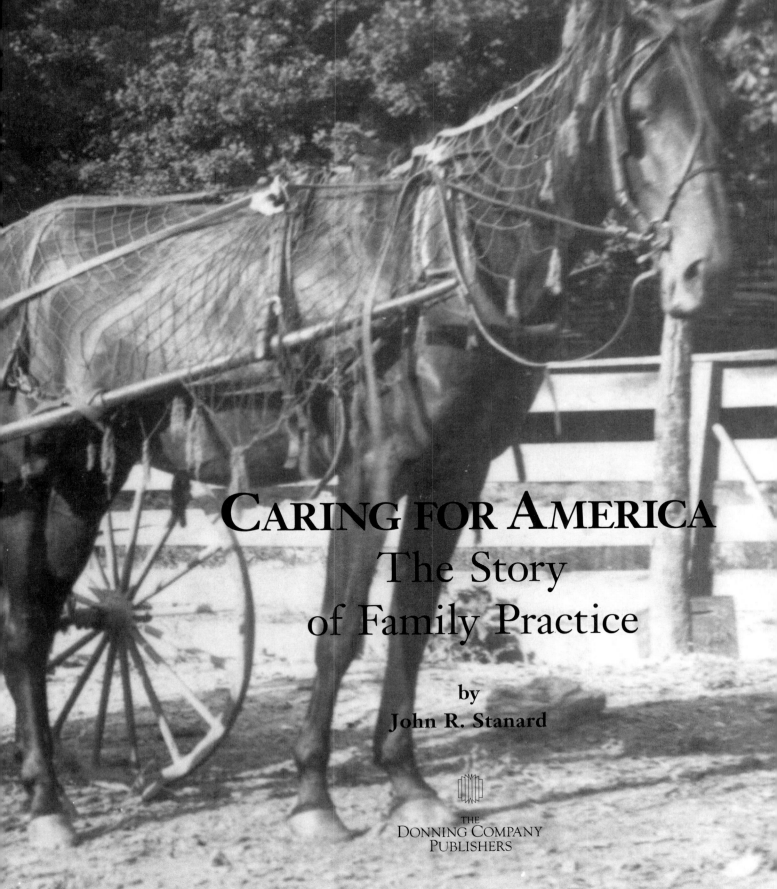

CARING FOR AMERICA
The Story
of Family Practice

by

John R. Stanard

THE
DONNING COMPANY
PUBLISHERS

*T*his book is dedicated to the memory of Fred L. Kneibert, M.D., the family doctor who delivered me; to Kenneth C. Li, M.D., who keeps me healthy now; and to all of America's family physicians—past, present and future.

J.R.S.

Horse and Buggy Doc

Title Pages: William Henderson Mayfield, M.D., stands beside his horse (wearing protective horsefly net) and buggy in Bollinger County, Mo., circa 1885. He founded Will Mayfield College in Marble Hill, Mo., and was a professor at the old St. Louis College of Physicians and Surgeons. (Mrs. Nelda Wilkinson.)

The Donning Company/Publishers
184 Business Park Drive, Suite 106
Virginia Beach, Va. 23462

Steve Mull, General Manager
Nancy Schneiderheinze, Project Director
Richard A. Horwege, Editor
Joseph C. Schnellmann, Graphic Designer
Dawn V. Kofroth, Production Manager
Tony Lillis, Director of Marketing
Teri S. Arnold, Marketing Assistant

Library of Congress Cataloging-in-Publication Data:

Stanard, John R., 1940–
        Caring for America : the story of family practice / by John R. Stanard.
                    p.   cm.
        Includes bibliographical references and index.
        ISBN 0-89865-992-2 (alk. paper)
        1. Family medicine—United States.   I. Title.
R729.5.G4S68   1997
616—dc21
97-1850

                CIP

Printed in the United States of America

CONTENTS

FOREWORD 7

PREFACE AND ACKNOWLEDGMENTS 9

CHAPTER 1
Hippocrates: Father of Family Medicine 12

CHAPTER 2
The Fall and Rise of the Family Doctor 26

CHAPTER 3
Caring for America in 1997 49

CHAPTER 4
Training Physicians for the Specialty 108

CHAPTER 5
Leading Generalism Into the 21st Century 118

BIBLIOGRAPHY 124

INDEX 125

ABOUT THE AUTHOR 128

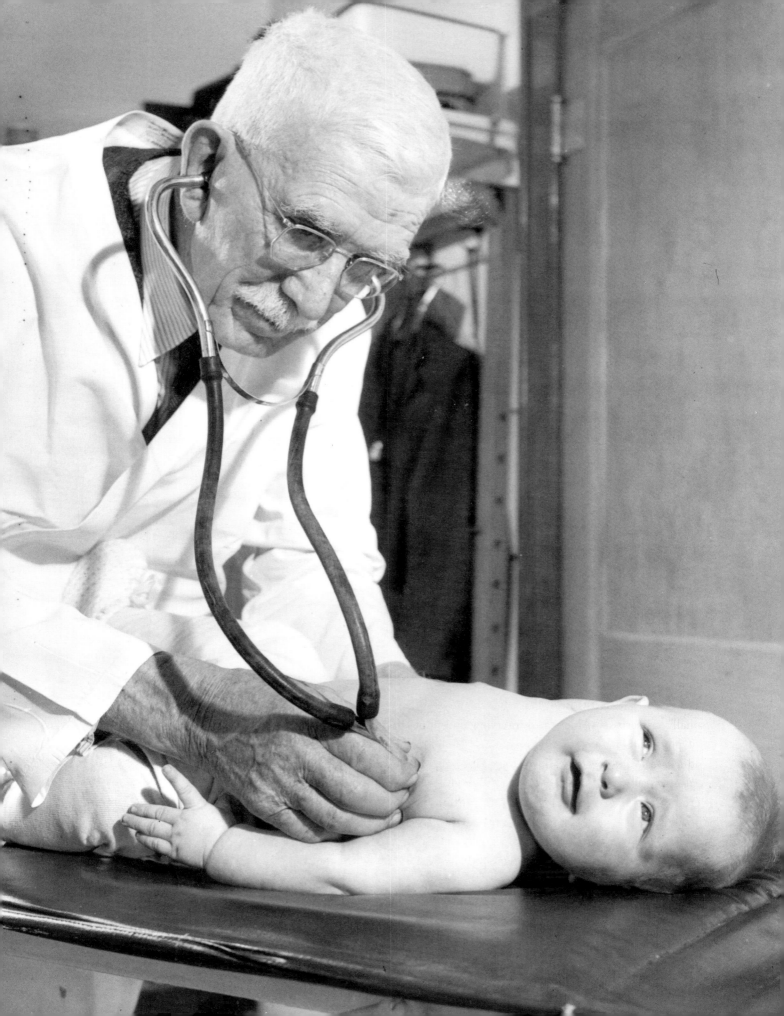

FOREWORD

his book commemorates and celebrates an event that happened 50 years ago when I was just a small boy, an event that would profoundly affect my life.

Meeting in Atlantic City, N.J., on June 10, 1947, a group of about 200 general practitioners (GPs) established the American Academy of General Practice, the predecessor of today's American Academy of Family Physicians, of which I am the 1996–97 president. The Academy's founders were facing a crisis in American medicine, which was increasingly dominated by limited specialists who weren't trained to provide comprehensive, ongoing care for patients and their families. There was a thinning of the ranks of GPs—and a growing lack of respect for GPs by others in American medicine. Those men in Atlantic City were fighting not only on behalf of America's families, who needed the GP's type of comprehensive care, but also for respect and for their economic lives.

The Academy grew quickly, and its leadership played a key role in eventually convincing organized medicine of the need for a new medical "specialty in breadth"—family practice—dedicated to the care of the patient in the context of the family and community. If those leaders had failed, I and thousands of men and women like me never would have had the opportunity to be trained and certified in this people-oriented specialty that I love.

There aren't enough pages in this book for great detail or to name every individual who played an important role along the way. The bibliography lists sources that can provide more information if you're interested.

One more point: This book's contents range from the old-fashioned to the modern, and so did the methods used to develop the book. The author personally crisscrossed America to interview and photograph the nine profiled family physicians—and research material was accessed via computer on the World Wide Web. This reminds me of family practice, which is built on the patient-centered traditions of general practice, with the benefit of today's high-powered technology and knowledge. May that marvelous blend of the old and the new help you achieve the best of health.

Patrick B. Harr, M.D.
1996–97 President
American Academy of Family Physicians

What's He Doing to Me?
Facing Page: Alfred M. Ridgway, M.D., age 82, examines an apprehensive baby in his Annandale, Minn., clinic in 1945. (Minneapolis Star-Journal-Tribune. *From Minnesota Historical Society.*)

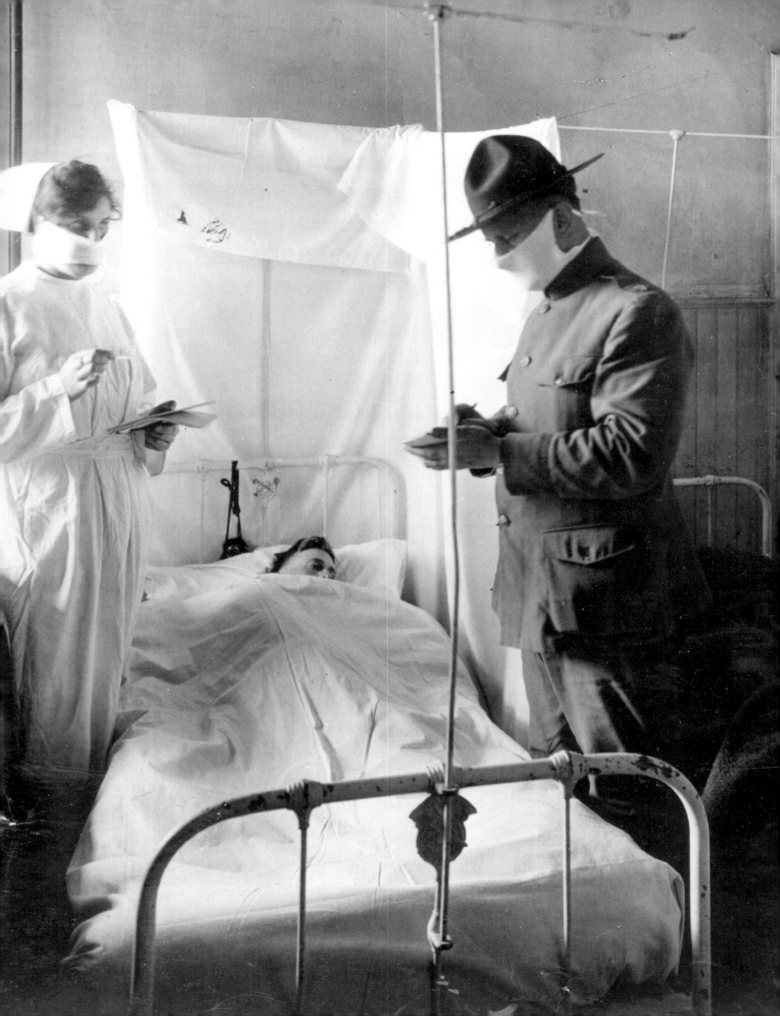

PREFACE AND ACKNOWLEDGMENTS

$\mathcal{T}$he prospect of producing this documentary history book on family physicians fascinated me from the beginning, when I heard that such a book would commemorate the 50th anniversary of the American Academy of Family Physicians (AAFP). As a photojournalist and newspaper editor, I already had developed a keen respect for the medical profession. That respect had deepened by the time I finished this book.

1996 was a challenging yet richly rewarding year for me, a time crammed full of new friends and interesting excursions into the far corners of our country. I traveled nearly 21,000 miles across America, shooting more than 1,600 color images to record the activities of nine family physicians.

David Baines, M.D., an American Indian, invited me to a sacred sweat lodge ceremony one cool evening in the heart of the Coeur d'Alene Reservation in Northwest Idaho. In the tropical heat of Kissimmee, Fla., John Hartman, M.D., and his gracious wife, Cleta, fed me wonderful food as I got acquainted with them and two of their delightful daughters.

In Mesa, Ariz., Leland Fairbanks, M.D., and his friends took me to restaurants that were smoke-free because of their work in the Arizonans Concerned About Smoking organization.

David McRay, M.D., jostled me in his four-wheel-drive Bronco to a promontory atop rugged Pine Mountain, where we watched the sun set over his East Tennessee community of Jellico.

Sister Roseanne Cook, M.D., a saint disguised as a Roman Catholic nun, showed me the "third world" living conditions of her impoverished black patients in Wilcox County, Ala. In the Ozark Mountains, I quickly discovered why "Dr. Tommy" Macdonnell, M.D., is so beloved in his hometown of Marshfield, Mo., where his father practiced before him.

Neil Calman, M.D., took me to exotic restaurants and showed me the sights of New York City, where he operates the Institute for Urban Family Health and oversees the care of thousands of underserved patients. In Salt Lake City, Silvia Corral, M.D., daughter of Mexican-American farm workers, welcomed me into her home and demonstrated how she cares for three young children as a single mother, and still operates a clinic for homeless people.

Masked Against Flu
Facing Page: U.S. Army physician and Red Cross nurse wear masks on Nov. 19, 1918, during the epidemic of Spanish influenza, as they make rounds at the Fort Porter, N.Y., general hospital eight days after the World War I armistice was signed. (American Red Cross.)

Evelyn Lewis, M.D., a U.S. Navy medical officer, allowed me to shadow her at the Uniformed Services University of the Health Sciences in Bethesda, Md., where she teaches, sees patients and promotes racial diversity.

In addition, a genial Jack Colwill, M.D., longtime chairman of the Department of Family and Community Medicine at the University of Missouri–Columbia School of Medicine, helped me learn how family doctors are trained as he explained his school's well-known family practice residency program. And three of Colwill's residents—Mark Schabbing, M.D.; Jim Elam, M.D.; and Shane Foster, M.D.—allowed me to accompany them as they went about their business of learning to be family physicians.

I am indebted to my wife, Vida Loberg Stanard, for her steady encouragement and keen editorial judgment as she pores over the many drafts of my writing. As my first and toughest editor, she knows what I am trying to say even when I fail. She gently tells me, and that helps me finally get it right.

I extend my thanks to all the physicians and their patients who tolerated my cameras and questions. I appreciate the help of the AAFP staff, especially news editor Paula Haas Binder, who helped me locate many candidates for the profiles in this book, guided me through the project and skillfully edited and reworked my copy. Angela Curran, curator of the Archives for Family Practice of the AAFP Foundation, helped me immensely by providing research materials.

Dolores Shearon, medical news coordinator at the University of Missouri–Columbia School of Medicine, suggested good candidates for the profiles section and helped in many other ways. Kathy Wolpers Sanders, interim librarian at the University of Arkansas at Little Rock, assisted me with a computer-based search for articles on family practice. Curators and librarians at more than 40 other institutions and societies helped me locate historical medical images.

Thomas Rockwell, son of famed artist Norman Rockwell, shared with me his personal recollections of the family doctor who was the subject of his father's painting and sketches on pages 100 and 101.

Finally, I appreciate the confidence and support of Nancy Schneiderheinze of Donning Company/Publishers, who recommended me for this project.

For those of you who are interested, I shot the modern photographs in the book with two 35mm cameras: a 25-year-old Nikon F Photomic FTN and a newer Nikon F-3HP. My lenses, all Nikkor, were the 24mm F2, the 55mm F1.2, the 85mm F1.4 and the 135mm F2.8. The film was Fuji 800 Super G Plus and Kodak Ektapress 1600, rated normally and shot entirely with available light.

John R. Stanard

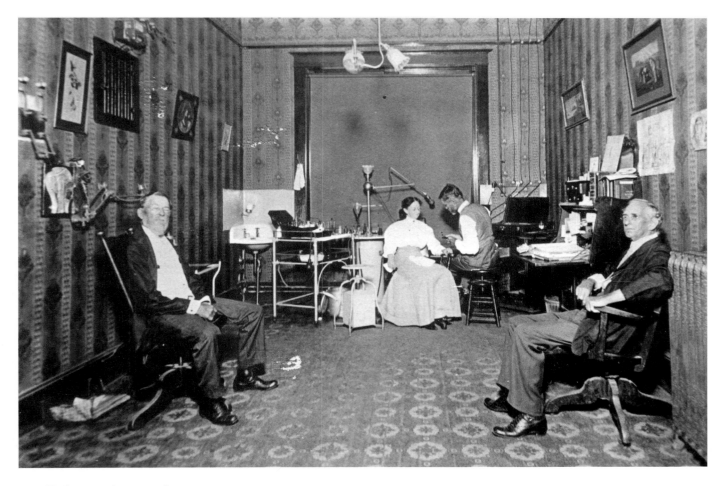

Privacy, Anyone?

Dr. J.G. Dorsey cares for a female patient in his combination office/waiting room in Wichita, Kan., circa 1911, while two men wait. Dorsey was born in Virginia, graduated from the Keokuk Medical College and was a general practitioner in north Missouri before moving to Wichita in the 1890s and specializing in eye surgery. (William J. Smither, M.D.)

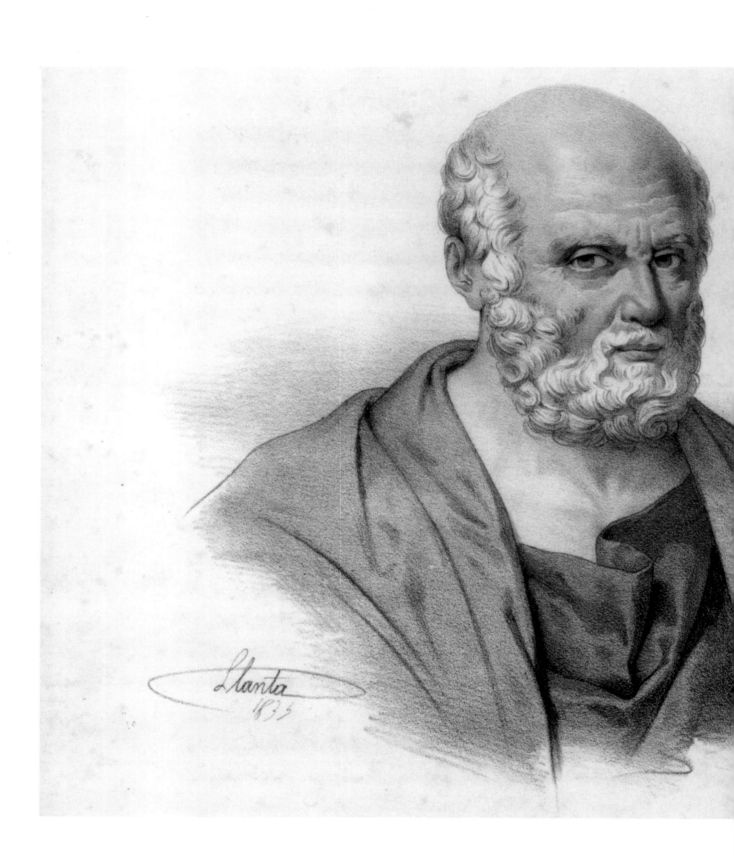

Llanta
1835

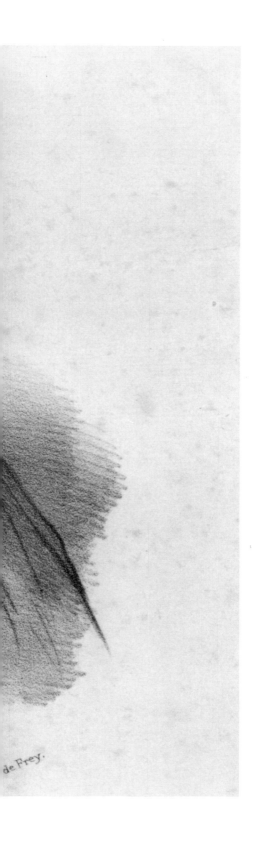

CHAPTER 1

Hippocrates: Father of Family Medicine

*I*n 1969, swept along by a torrent of public outcry for better, more accessible medical care and responding to its own perception that change was indeed necessary, American medicine established its 20th specialty: family practice, the "specialty in breadth." It was the first new specialty in 21 years.

The story of how and why family practice was established in America is full of color and controversy and the social upheavals of the 1960s. But the specialty's underpinnings go back much farther than the mid-20th century.

To trace the earliest roots of family practice, one has to go back in time, past all the astounding medical technology of today, beyond the landmark scientific discoveries of the previous century, back to the time of Hippocrates, the Father of Medicine and, in some ways, the Father of *Family* Medicine.

Before Hippocrates, superstition ruled. Though the ancients discovered some remarkable medical remedies, the actual causes of diseases—and successful treatments—were attributed to the supernatural. Elaborate ceremonies, even gruesome human sacrifice, often accompanied healing efforts

Hippocrates

Often called the Father of Medicine, Hippocrates arguably could be called the Father of Family Medicine as well. Though based on flimsy evidence, this 19th-century engraving is the universally accepted image of Hippocrates, who was born about 460 B.C. (Yale University, Harvey Cushing/John Hay Whitney Medical Library.)

13

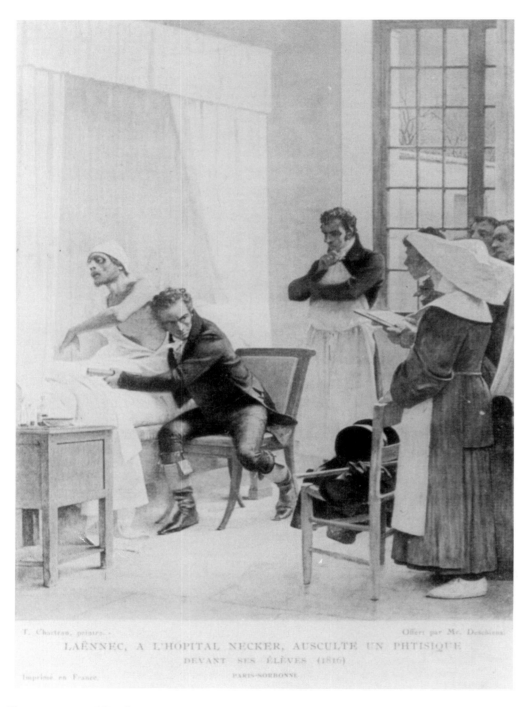

T. Chartran, peintre.   Offert par Mr. Deschiens.

LAËNNEC, A L'HOPITAL NECKER, AUSCULTE UN PHTISIQUE
DEVANT SES ÉLÈVES (1816)

Imprimé en France.   PARIS-SORBONNE

Laennec at Necker

French physician Rene Laennec, inventor of the stethoscope, listens to a man's chest with his ear.
He clutches in his left hand the first version (a tube of paper) of the instrument still in use today.
Laennec himself died of pulmonary tuberculosis in 1825. (Oil painting by T. Chartran.
Laennec Listening with His Ear Against the Chest of a Patient at Necker Hospital.
National Library of Medicine, Bethesda, Md.)

aimed at appeasing appropriate gods or driving away evil spirits.

Scientists have found trephined (punctured) skulls dating as far back as 10,000 years, along with the tools used to punch the holes. Modern surgeons still use the procedure to ease pressure on the brain in some cases. To relieve pain, early American Indians chewed willow bark, which contains salicin, a substance related to the salicylates in aspirin. By 2500 B.C., the Egyptians were treating fractures and wounds, and worshipping as their god of healing an earlier physician named Imhotep, the world's first doctor known by name.

But Hippocrates, born about 460 B.C. on the Greek island of Cos in the Aegean Sea, founded a school of thought that ignored the supernatural/medical consensus of his age. He wasn't opposed to religion—but he was opposed to nonrational magic.

Hippocrates believed that each disease had only natural causes and proceeded according to its natural order. Noted Yale University surgeon and medical historian Sherwin B. Nuland, M.D., in his *Doctors: The Biography of Medicine*, says: "This injunction to turn a blind eye to the possibility of a deity or mystical influence in the causes and treatment of disease was the greatest contribution made by the school of Hippocrates."

Hippocrates and his fellow practitioners focused totally on the patient and the patient's environment. They tried to assist nature in restoring the patient to

Dramatic Illustration
An engraving from Harper's Weekly *in 1860, titled* The Sick Woman in Bellevue Hospital, New York, Overrun by Rats, *showed the deplorable conditions in some of America's hospitals in the mid-19th century. (Wood engraving. National Library of Medicine, Bethesda, Md.)*

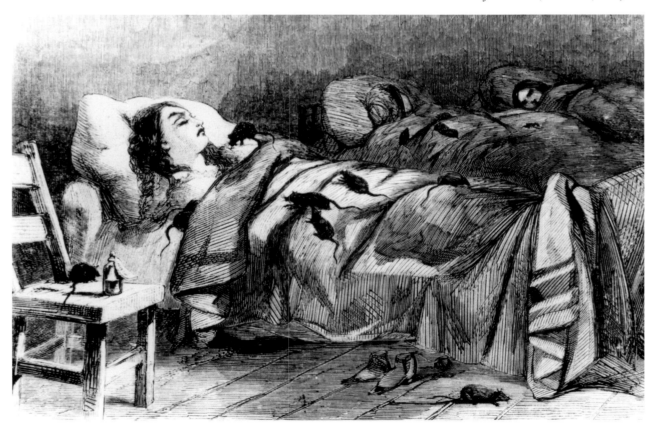

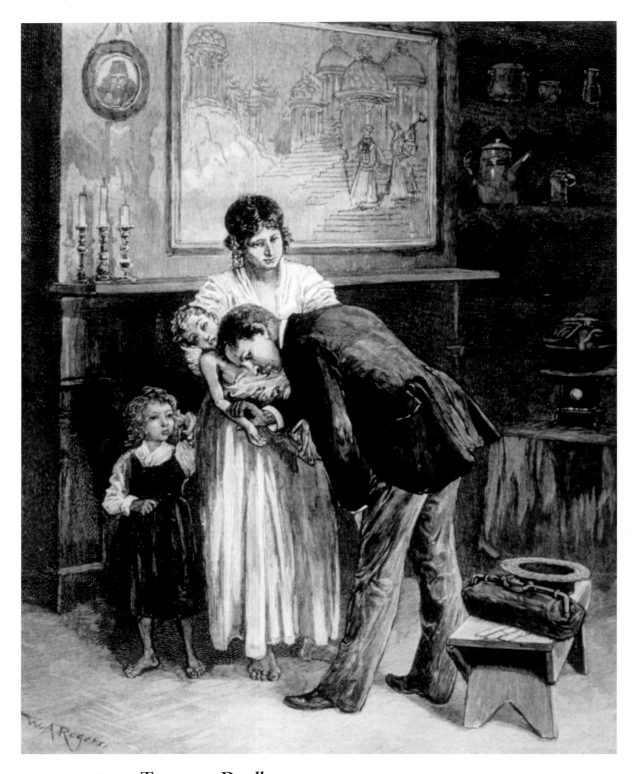

Tenement Dwellers
A New York City Board of Health doctor makes a visit to a mother and her children in a tenement building in this illustration from Harper's Weekly *on Aug. 10, 1889. (National Library of Medicine, Bethesda, Md.)*

a state of health, which they considered to be harmony, or the balance of forces, in the body.

This inclusive approach was apparent when Hippocrates wrote, "It is necessary for the physician to provide not only the needed treatment, but to provide for the patient himself, and those beside him, and for his outside affairs."

The approach lifted Greek medicine out of the mire of superstition and witchcraft—and made Hippocrates in many ways the Father of Family Medicine. He and his colleagues presaged America's general practitioners, those mainstays of the nation's health care for many decades of the early 20th century—and their heirs, today's family physicians, who combine the best aspects of general practice with postgraduate training across many medical fields and who practice with a focus on the entire patient in the context of the family and community.

With the decline of classical Greece and the rise of the Roman Empire, the Hippocratic teachings degenerated into many competing and illogical philosophies. The young Greek physician named Galen, born in A.D. 130, led medicine back to science, if not back to a focus on the patient as a whole. Considered the founder of experimental medicine, Galen studied writings about human cadaver dissections (which were usually forbidden in his time) and did extensive anatomical research on animals. As the surgeon for the town coliseum, he saw horribly injured gladiators with gaping wounds that revealed organs still functioning.

Yale's Nuland writes, "Galen's research into anatomy and physiology pointed the way to a new understanding of the body and how it gets sick."

Through the Middle Ages and the Renaissance, which saw a fourth of Europe die of bubonic plague and other epidemics, few medical advances were recorded. At last, late in the Renaissance, more breakthroughs occurred. Italian physician Andreas Vesalius wrote the first scientific text on human anatomy in 1543. His contemporary, French military surgeon Ambroise Paré, not only was the greatest surgeon of his time, but also wrote what became the standard surgical texts for centuries.

And still medical science advanced. In 1628, British physician William Harvey wrote about his discovery of the circulation of blood caused by the pumping action of the heart, which Nuland describes as "the greatest gift ever made by one man to the science and art of medicine."

In 1796, English physician Edward Jenner developed a safe inoculation against the dreaded smallpox. Recorded as the first known vaccination, it paved the way for immunology.

The 1800s saw many significant advances. In 1816, French physician Rene Laennec invented the stethoscope, an instrument still used universally by physicians around the world. In the 1840s, several American physicians,

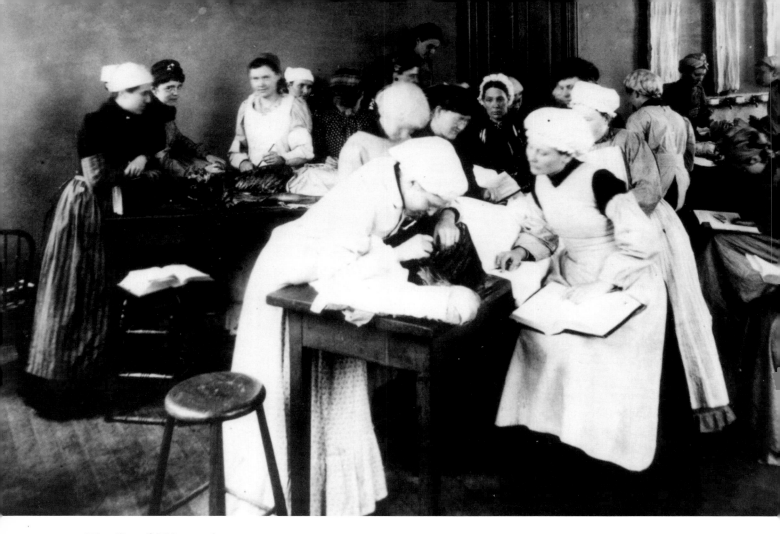

No Coed Dissection
Female medical students dissect cadavers in a University of Michigan anatomy class segregated by sex, circa 1891. (Bentley Historical Library, University of Michigan Medical School Records.)

A Chilling Effect
Medical students work on cadavers in the dissecting room at the State University of Iowa Medical School in 1889. W.A. Rohlf, M.D., is at left. The coats and hats probably indicate the room is cold. (State Historical Society of Iowa– Iowa City.)

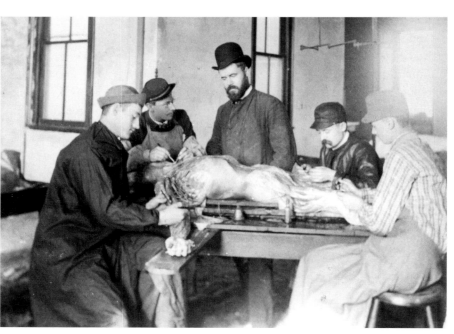

including John Collins Warren and Crawford Long, independently demonstrated the use of ether in painless surgery. Before that, surgery could be excruciatingly painful, even with the use of opiate and alcoholic sedatives.

In 1847, Ignaz Semmelweis, a young obstetrician at Vienna General Hospital, discovered that 10 times more mothers were dying of childbed fever in one ward than in another. Students and teachers, who worked on putrid cadavers every day, delivered all the babies in the first ward. Midwives delivered all the infants in the other. When thorough hand-washing with a chlorine solution was ordered for the students and teachers, the death rate in their ward dropped to just over 1 percent, the same as in the midwives' ward. Thus Semmelweis was able to offer a theory based on the spread of bacterial contamination years before French chemist Louis Pasteur and German physician Robert Koch established the germ theory of disease.

Aided by improved microscopes, scientists by the end of the 1800s had identified the microbes that cause many infectious diseases. And Rudolf Virchow, a giant of German science and medicine, would become known as the founder of pathology, the study of the nature of disease.

A monumental discovery came in 1865 from British surgeon Joseph Lister, who drastically reduced death rates from wound infection from 46 percent to 15 percent by using carbolic acid as an antiseptic on incisions. His theory led to the modern practice of aseptic surgery, in which wounds are protected from germs.

After the discoveries of X-rays and radium in the 1890s, the 20th century ushered in a dazzling array of scientific medical advances, many of them in the United States. Among these have been sulfa drugs and antibiotics in the 1930s and '40s, polio vaccines in the '50s and '60s and astounding, ongoing improvements in organ transplants, surgical techniques and diagnostic imaging technology.

And so the science of medicine marched brilliantly forward, seducing many in medicine to believe that all illnesses could be reduced to the lowest common denominator: biological causes. Medicine fell in love with biomedical technology; the union eventually led to medicine's fragmentation into specialty fiefdoms, most focusing on a new technological tool or a specific organ system—not on the *patient* in the context of family and environment. The resulting armory of treatments often succeeded with biologically caused conditions, but it had limited success in such areas as preventing disease by promoting a healthy lifestyle. Witness the rise in obesity, tobacco use and unprotected sex, which has led to such modern-day plagues as heart disease, cancer and AIDS.

Medicine's infatuation with technology also caused many to see the *art* of medicine—the role of the physician as a healer in a personal relationship with the patient—as a poor substitute for knowledge, and the province of pretenders and exploiters.

Hippocrates would have wept.

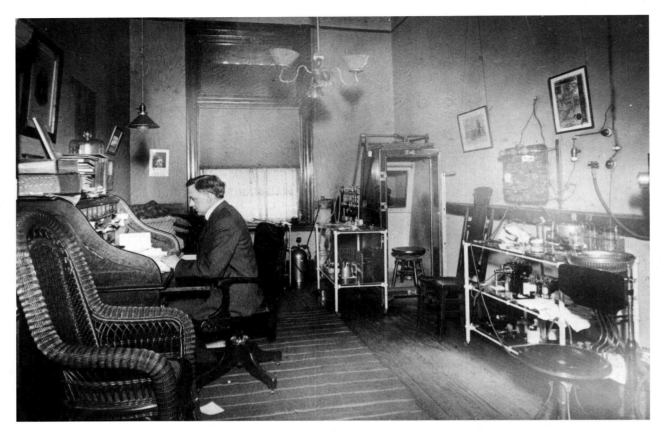

A Century Ago

H. Longstreet Taylor, M.D., works in his office in St. Paul, Minn., in 1886.
(Flash-Lighters of Minneapolis. Minnesota Historical Society.)

A Scientific Approach

William Talley, M.D., of Marble Hill, Mo., and his compound microscope, circa 1887. He was among the first physicians in the region to accept Pasteur's germ theory. Talley graduated from the St. Louis Medical College in 1868. He paid $700 for the microscope, using it to diagnose diseases in his backwoods area of the Missouri Ozarks. (Mrs. Nelda Wilkinson.)

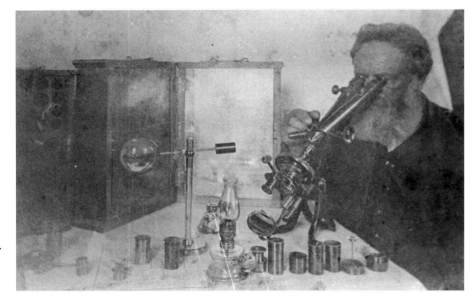

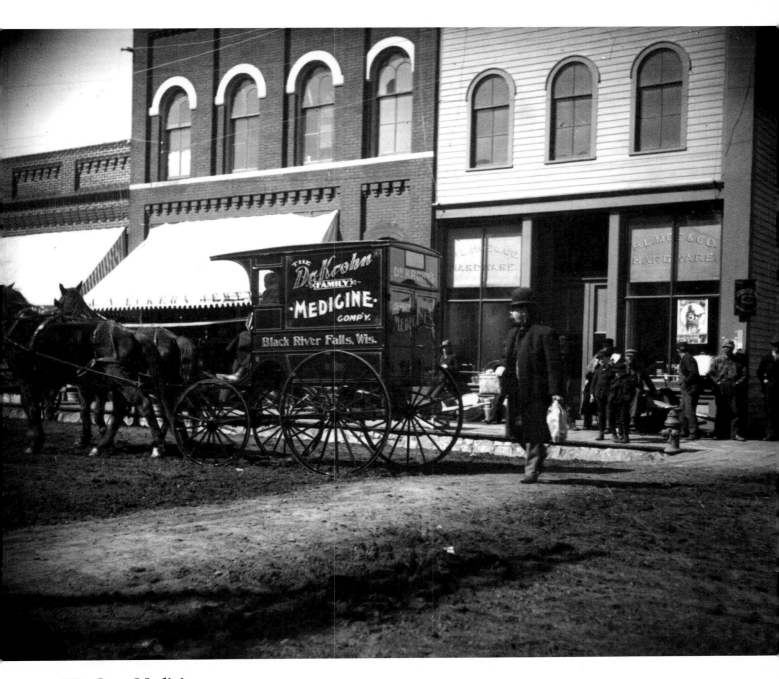

His Own Medicine

Dr. Eugene Krohn drives the Krohn Family Medicine Company wagon along a street in Black River Falls, Wis., near the turn of the century. Krohn was described as a "first-rate general practitioner and skillful surgeon." He also owned a drugstore and operated a patent medicine business. (State Historical Society of Wisconsin. WHi {V2} 62.)

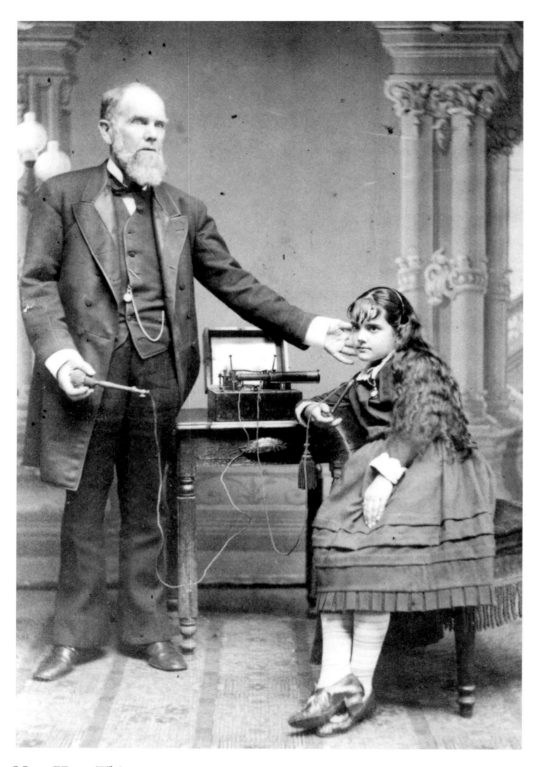

Now Hear This
Dr. J.K. Rickey uses a device to test a small girl's hearing, somewhere in Iowa, circa
1900. (State Historical Society of Iowa–Iowa City.)

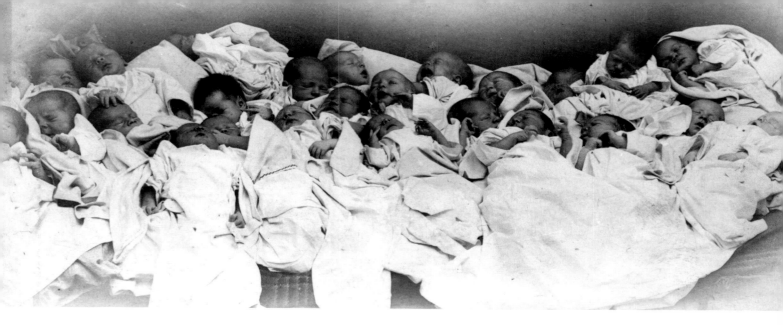

A Baby Picture

The nursery at Boston's Lying In Hospital had at least 25 babies on hand in 1899 when a photographer piled them up and made this picture. (The Francis A. Countway Library of Medicine, Harvard Medical School.)

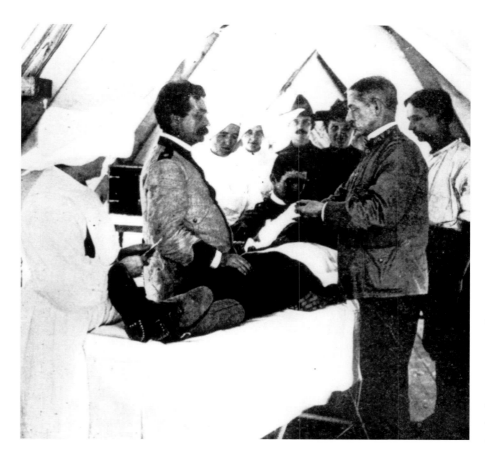

War Casualty

A U.S. Army physician treats a soldier wounded during the Spanish-American War in 1898. The soldier had been returned to a military hospital at Montauk, N.Y. (National Library of Medicine, Bethesda, Md.)

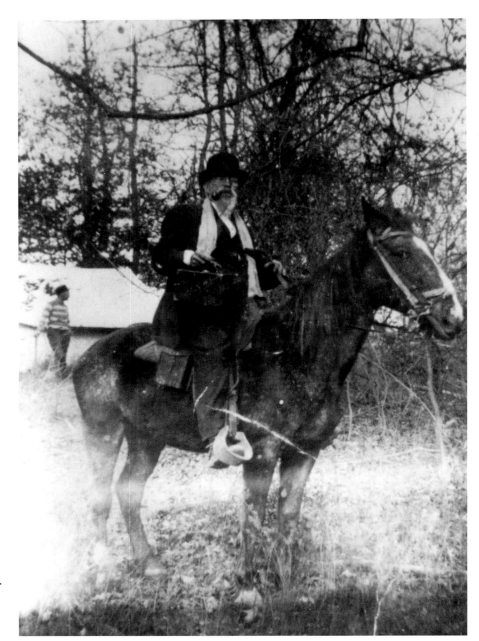

Doc Holliday

Dr. Milton J. Holliday was a circuit-riding physician who covered a 10-mile radius on horseback from his Butler County, Mo., home in the late 1800s and early 1900s. Granddaughter Mildred Perkins remembers that he "went when he was needed, whether they had money or not. Everybody owed grandpa when he died in 1923." (Mildred Perkins.)

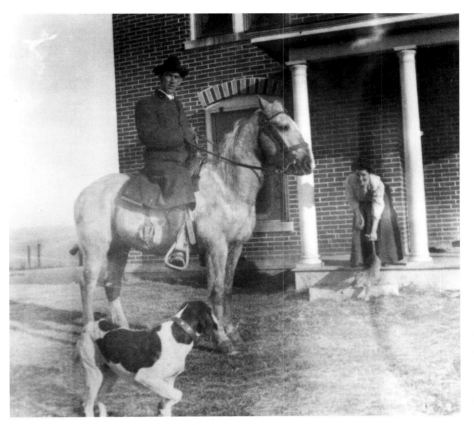

The Cat Stayed Home

F.B. Farrington, M.D., leaves his home at Greentop, Mo., to make a house call on horseback in 1908. He is accompanied by his hunting dog, Bob. Farrington's sister-in-law, Merdal Edwards, grabs the family cat's tail to keep it away from the dog. Dr. Farrington graduated in 1905 from St. Louis University after nine years of college education. (Missouri State Archives.)

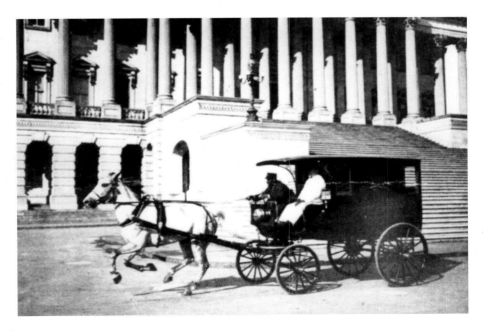

An Emergency Run

A horse-drawn ambulance from the Central Dispensary and Emergency Hospital races past the Capitol Building in Washington, D.C., in 1906. (National Library of Medicine, Bethesda, Md.)

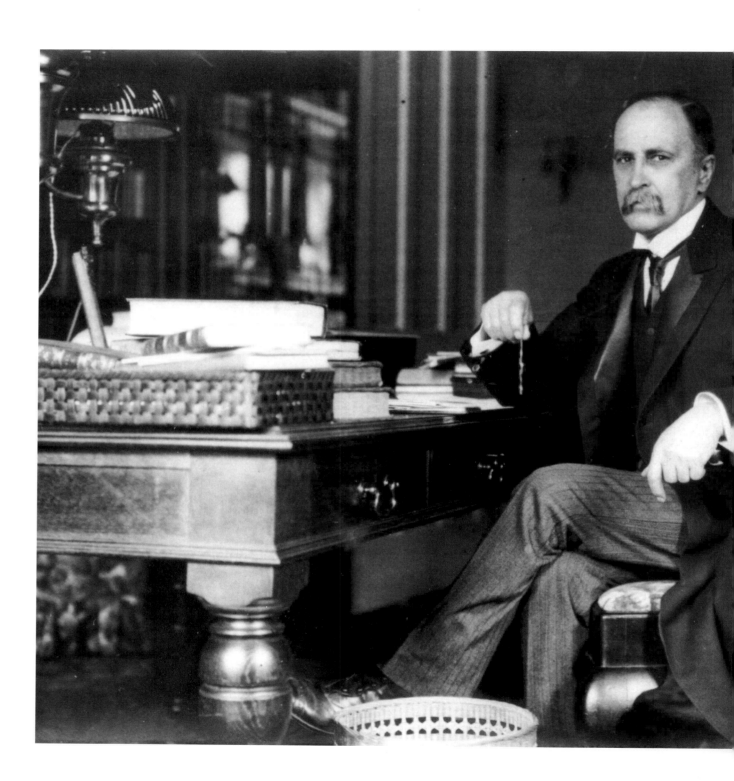

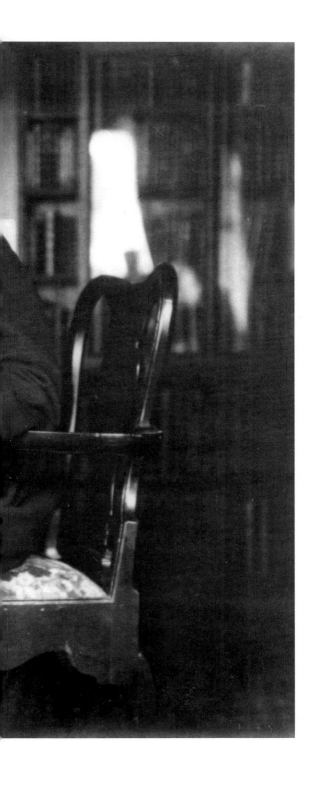

CHAPTER 2

The Fall and Rise of the Family Doctor

*D*espite astounding scientific progress, American medicine was in a sorry state in the last quarter of the 19th century. While there were good physicians who did the best they could with the knowledge they had, many aspiring doctors without even a high school diploma were admitted to substandard medical schools. They began their practices after only minimal training and abbreviated apprenticeships under mentors of dubious qualifications. Hospitals were filthy, and many well-known practitioners still were skeptical about the proven Listerian concept of aseptic surgery.

It was estimated that about half of America's leading physicians born between 1840 and 1890 studied in Germanic medical schools, at least 10,000 of them in Vienna in the 45 years following 1870. Only Baltimore's Johns Hopkins, opened in 1893, could compare with its Teutonic counterparts.

After a study of 155 U.S. and Canadian medical schools

Revered Physician

Sir William Osler, M.D., world-famous doctor and teacher of clinical medicine, at his desk in the early 1900s. He was a founder of the Johns Hopkins University School of Medicine. His text, Principles and Practices of Medicine, *was reprinted for the 15th time in 1947, 28 years after his death. (Yale University, Harvey Cushing/John Hay Whitney Medical Library.)*

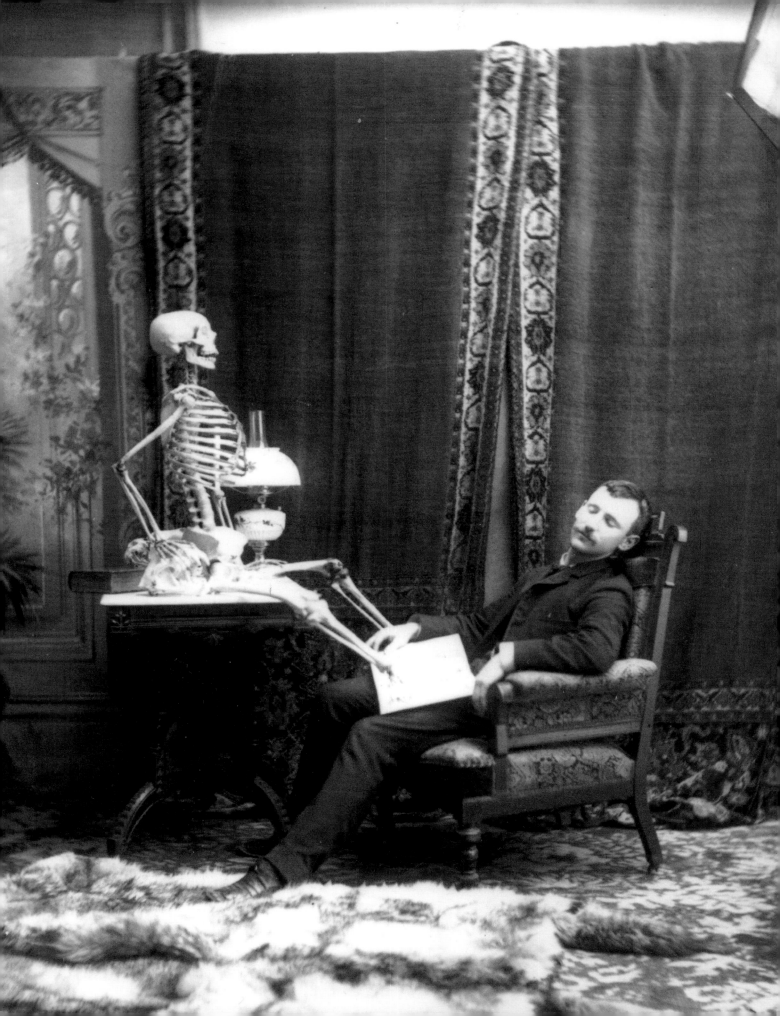

commissioned by the Carnegie Foundation, educator/investigator Abraham Flexner delivered a scathing report in 1910. He found faculties were poorly trained, and standards were low. Profits were the top priority of the owners, who usually were the professors. Johns Hopkins was singled out as a notable exception. Five other schools were given a passing grade, but they were classed far below Johns Hopkins.

Marginal medical schools were closed in droves. Flexner was put in charge of a $600 million fund created by American philanthropists to elevate medical training. As he would say later, he helped guide the rise of American medical education "from the lowest status to the highest in the civilized world."

In the years after the Flexner revolution, most graduates of America's improved medical schools went into general practice, providing their enhanced skills in surgery, maternity care, care of children and other fields to people throughout the nation. They delivered most of the babies, and maternal and infant mortality rates dropped sharply as care improved. Through dedication to their patients' continuing care every day, these general practitioners (GPs) established a public image that remains symbolic of what people expect from their physicians. And people could reasonably expect to get this kind of care: In 1930, about 80 percent of American physicians were GPs; only 20 percent were specialists.

But times changed. During the 1940s, economic pressures and the explosion of medical information continued the fragmentation of medicine into limited specialties and sparked the decline of general practice.

Many medical students chose to become specialists to feel more secure in knowing almost everything about a limited area or organ system. They also were influenced by their professors, most of whom were themselves specialists. The faulty assumption grew that the generalist physician required less training and was therefore less important than the specialist.

The death knell for general practice began with World War II. The U.S.

Boning Up On His Books
Facing Page: Trinidad, Colo., photographer Oliver E. Aultman, known for clowning with his subjects, made this posed photograph in his studio, circa 1890. The subject asleep with his book and skeleton likely is a medical student. (Colorado Historical Society, Neg. F37832.)

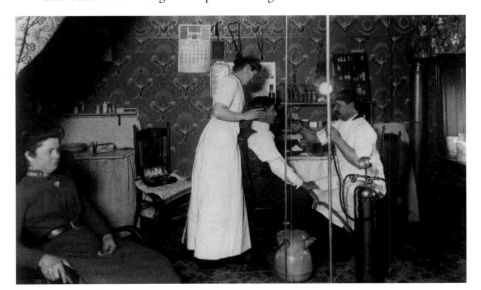

Treatment in Kansas
Dr. R.E. Gray, right, treats a patient with some type of gas in his office at Garden City, Kan., in January of 1901. A nurse assists him while a family member waits. (Kansas State Historical Society.)

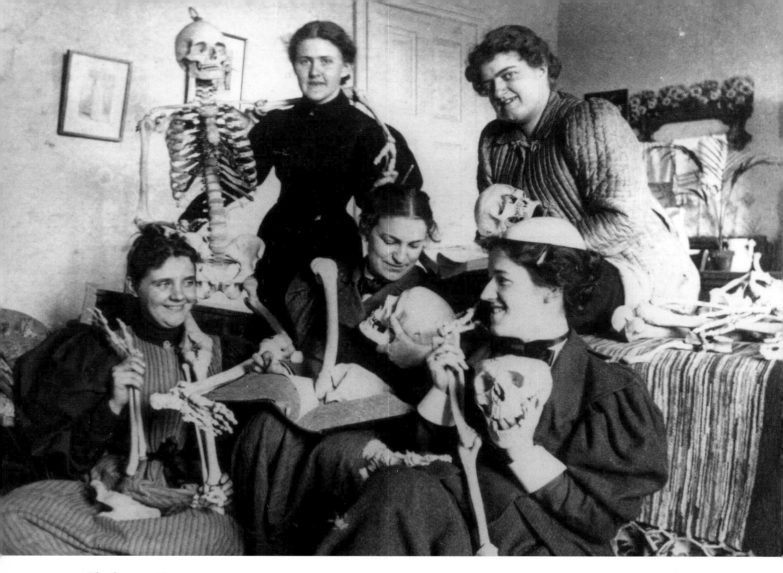

Skeleton Crew

Students at the Woman's Medical College of Pennsylvania in Philadelphia clown around with their study skeletons, circa 1895. (Archives and Special Collections on Women in Medicine, Allegheny University of the Health Sciences.)

First Hospital

A young resident physician treats a female child, as nurses observe, in the outpatient service area of Pennsylvania Hospital in Philadelphia, circa 1893. The institution was founded in 1751 as America's first hospital. (Pennsylvania Hospital, Philadelphia.)

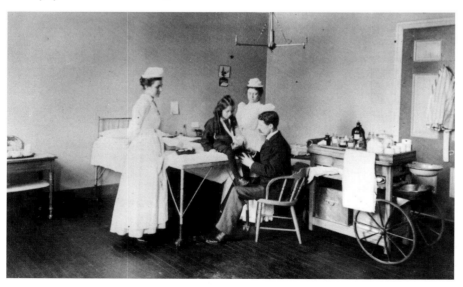

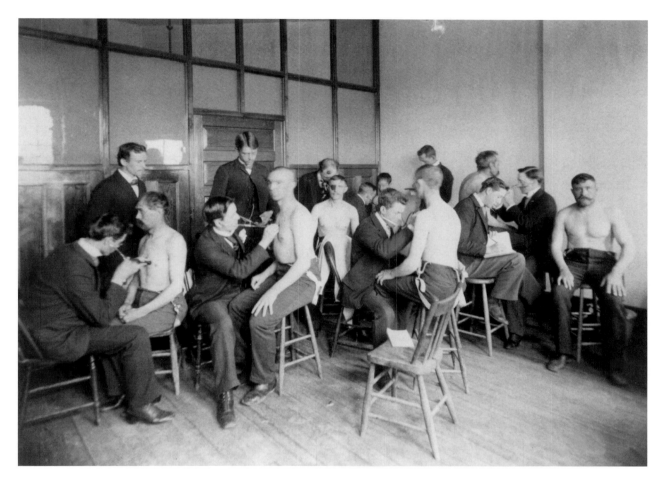

Congress approved military exemptions for medical students after graduation—provided they went into residency training. But there were no residencies in general practice.

Furthermore, many military hospitals were set up by specialists, who wanted more specialists to staff them. In some cases, specialists on staff at a civilian hospital were transported as a unit to serve together in a military hospital. These hospitals were located miles from the battle lines or in cities. The armed forces also gave greater rank and therefore higher pay and prestige to specialists.

General practitioners, with lower rank, pay, and prestige, ducked bullets and cared for the walking wounded on the front lines. The result, not surprisingly, was a rush of medical graduates into specialty residencies.

After the war's end in 1945, the GI Bill paid allowances for medical school and up to four years of residency training—but there still were no general practice residencies. In addition, the American College of Surgeons, at the time the only agency that accredited hospitals, decided to no longer allow GPs to perform surgical procedures in hospitals—procedures that the GPs had performed before military service.

Learning to Listen
Male medical students practice auscultation on each other with stethoscopes at the University of Michigan Medical School, circa 1893. (Bentley Historical Library, University of Michigan Medical School Records.)

31

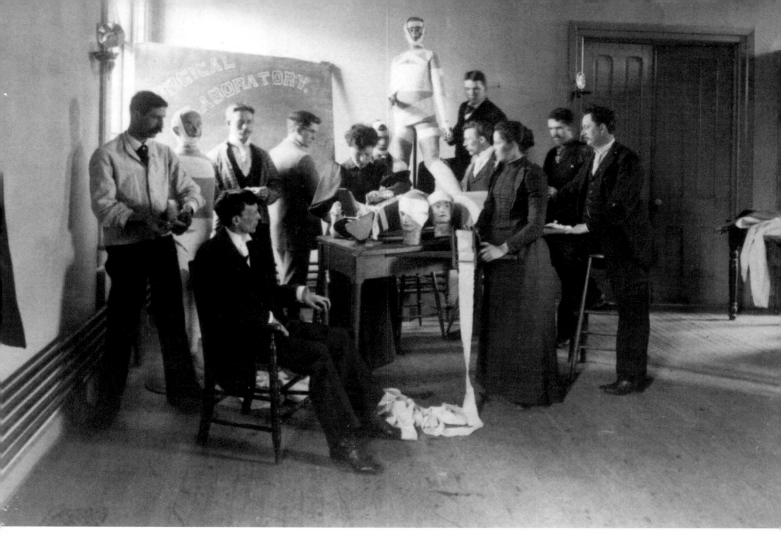

Perfecting Techniques

University of Michigan medical students practice bandaging and fracture dressing techniques, circa 1893. The sign in left background says "Surgical Laboratory." (Bentley Historical Library, University of Michigan Medical School Records.)

Arkansas Colleagues

Monroe D. McClain, M.D., right, sits at his desk and visits with colleague C.C. Reed, M.D., in his Little Rock office in February of 1909. McClain died two years later in an automobile accident, one of Arkansas' first traffic fatalities, according to his son, Monroe D. McClain Jr., M.D. The younger McClain, who was 86 in 1996, is a retired family physician in Little Rock. (Historical Research Center, University of Arkansas for Medical Sciences Library, Little Rock.)

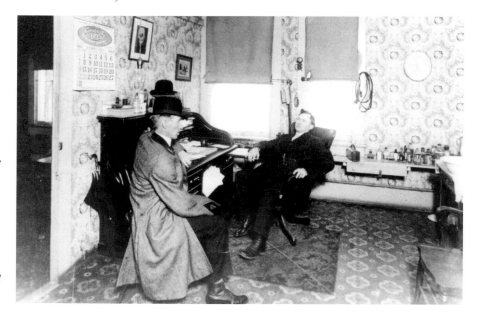

It's no surprise that specialty residencies burgeoned from about 5,200 in 1940 to 22,000 in 1952, creating a swell of specialists who poured out into civilian practice.

General practice gradually hit bottom, becoming a "last man's club" of sorts, and the GP's type of medical care—centering on the whole patient in the context of the family and environment—was fast becoming lost in the specialist shuffle.

General practitioners began to be in short supply, and health care was becoming depersonalized and expensive—and unavailable to many since most specialists located in cities, close to hospitals. As the static population of GPs aged, many smaller communities lost their physicians.

Those GPs who remained had to fight back, not only for respect but also for their economic lives. At their insistence, the American Medical Association in 1945 authorized a section on general practice, providing GPs with a voice in the AMA's policymaking body. In 1947, GPs established their own national society, the American Academy of General Practice (AAGP). Now, family doctors could make their voices heard in organized medicine.

By 1950, the AAGP had 10,000 members. The rapid growth was fueled in part by the high standards the Academy established: Each member was required to complete 150 hours of continuing medical education every three years to retain membership.

Efforts accelerated to create more general practice residencies, but few chose the training because there was no established, codified body of knowledge for general practice, and because the residencies were perceived by many to lead nowhere. In contrast, those who completed specialty residency training could become "board certified" by passing an examination offered by their field's certifying body. So to many GPs, the logical answer to the predicament seemed to be the creation of a board certification process for a new "specialty in breadth" that would become the heir of general practice: family practice.

For years, politics delayed the development of this new specialty: There was opposition both from the existing specialties *and* from within the ranks of GPs themselves. After all, for many GPs, specialties had been "the enemy" for so long, it was difficult to consider becoming one! And some GPs who still performed major surgery feared they'd have to give it up if they became certified in the new specialty.

The debate, and attempts to create better, more popular GP residencies, continued through the 1950s and most of the '60s. But external forces in the '60s gave the family practice movement the impetus it needed. The Medicare bill was signed into law in 1965, but even with this improved access to care for some Americans, many found it increasingly difficult to find doctors to care for themselves and their families. In addition, the rising social consciousness of young people—which also led to the sexual revolution and to protests against the Vietnam War—created idealistic medical students who believed strongly in the concept of personalized, comprehensive care.

While many general practitioners had been using this comprehensive approach for years, experience—not specific training—led them to it. Many medical leaders in the '60s, including those in the American Academy of General Practice, became convinced that specialty status, solid residency training and a certification examination would be the key elements in attracting more medical students to generalism.

The year 1966 was a high point in the drive for a new specialty:

• The National Commission on Community Health Services, established by the American Public Health Association and the National Health Council, issued a report (called the Folsom Report, or the Harvard Report) asserting, "Every individual should have a personal physician who is the central point for integration and continuity of all medical . . . services to his patient. Such a physician will emphasize the practice of preventive medicine. . . . He will be aware of the many and varied social, emotional and environmental factors that influence the health of his patient and his patient's family. . . . His concern will be for the patient as a whole, and his relationship with the patient must be a continuing one."

• The Citizens Commission on Graduate Medical Education (the Millis Commission), an external body established at the AMA's request, called for a physician who "focuses not upon individual organs and systems but upon the whole man, who lives in a complex social setting, and . . . knows that diagnosis or treatment of a part often overlooks major causative factors and therapeutic opportunities."

• Finally, the Ad Hoc Committee on Education for Family Practice (the Willard Committee), appointed by the AMA Council on Medical Education, stated that the American public "does want and need a large number of well-qualified family physicians." It further recommended that training should include extensive experiences simulating a family-oriented medical practice—a drastic change from the hospital-based training of other specialties.

On February 8, 1969, after a great deal of effort on the part of the AAGP, the AMA, and other bodies, the Liaison Committee for Specialty Boards finally approved family practice, the new "specialty in breadth."

The new specialty's certifying board, the American Board of Family Practice (ABFP), offered its first certification exam in 1970. The process of rebuilding the ranks of personal physicians who would care for America had begun. And Americans desperately needed these new specialists: Within a few years, only 20 percent of the nation's physicians were general practitioners.

No GPs were "grandfathered" into board-certified status, something that had occurred in other specialties when their boards were established. Instead, GPs were allowed to sit for the examination via the "practice-eligible" route and had to pass the full exam, just as residency-trained family physicians would in ensuing years.

The ABFP also was the first specialty board to require that physicians pass a recertification exam every seven years in order to remain board certified.

In 1971, the American Academy of General Practice changed its name to the American Academy of Family Physicians.

The new specialty grew quickly. By 1975, there were 3,720 family practice residents studying in 250 programs approved by the Residency Review Committee for Family Practice. By 1985, the number of residents had doubled. By 1996, the total number of residency graduates topped 46,000.

As America approaches the 21st century, family practice has come into its own as the fastest-growing specialty in the United States. In 1996, it became the first specialty with residencies in all 50 states, with more than 10,100 residents in 452 programs. That year, membership in the American Academy of Family Physicians hit a record 83,000—including nearly 19,000 medical student members who are considering a future as a family physician.

Today's family physicians provide comprehensive, high-quality care in any medical environment, whether it's a health maintenance organization, a rural practice or anything in between. Their outlook centers on the patient in the context of the family and the community. They share a unique and personal relationship with their patients that's built on trust, and they serve as their patients' advocate and guide in the nation's evolving health care system.

Hippocrates would be proud.

A Pressure Check

Dr. William C. Thompson takes the blood pressure of a reclining patient in his office in Dublin, Ga., circa 1911. (Georgia Department of Archives and History.)

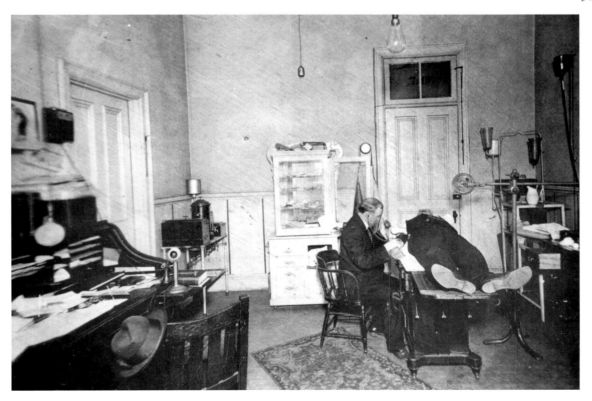

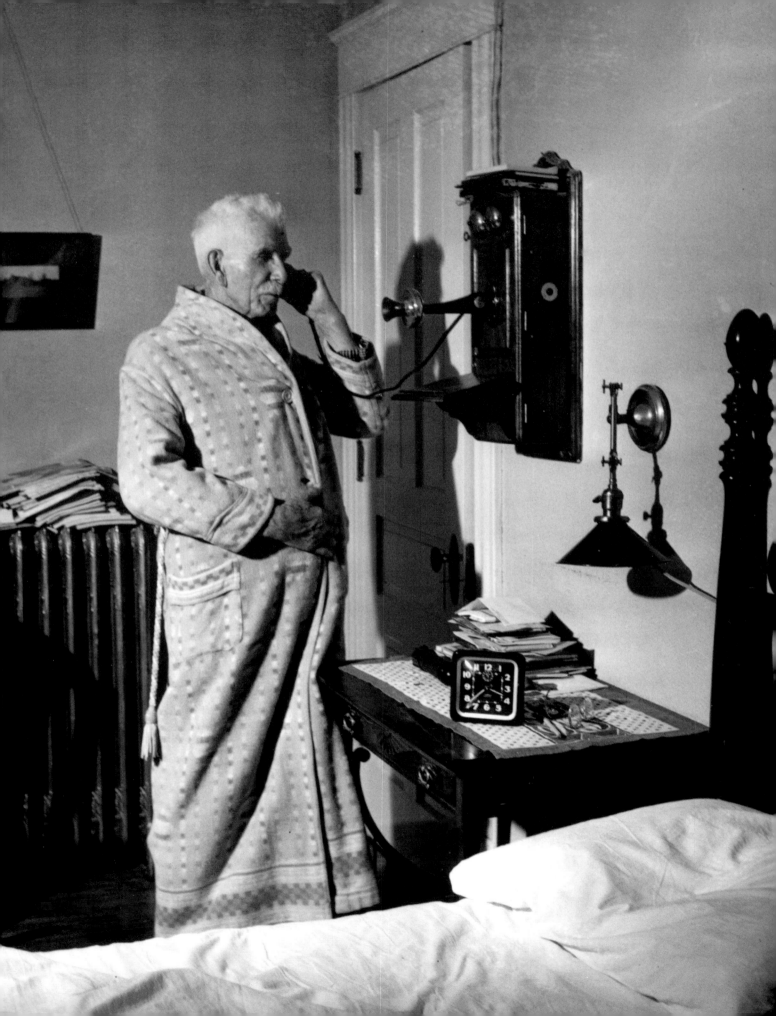

Six Decades of Practice

Alfred M. Ridgway, M.D., earned a medical degree from the University of Minnesota in 1890. He began practice that year in Annandale, west of Minneapolis. A biography written in 1914 reported Ridgway had "eight driving horses and two automobiles necessary to reach patients in his large rural practice." He was still working in 1945, at age 82, when a Minneapolis newspaper published a photo essay about him. (*Minneapolis Star-Journal-Tribune*, Minnesota Historical Society.)

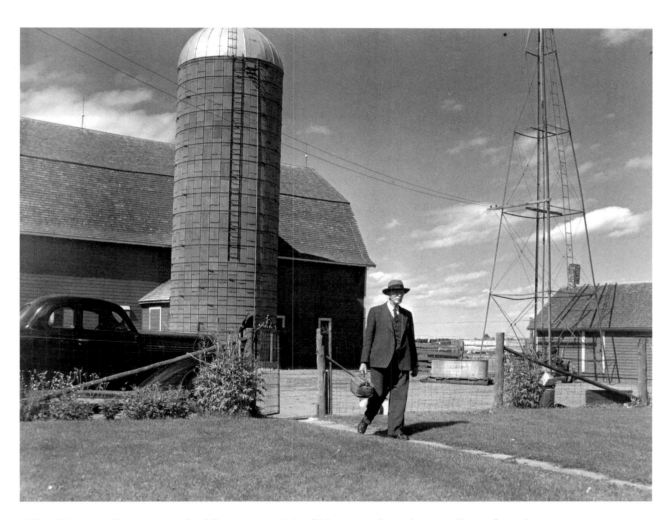

After driving miles out onto the Minnesota prairie, Ridgway makes a house call to a farm home.

Facing Page: *Ridgway starts his day at 3:37 a.m. when the telephone awakens him. It's a patient asking that he make a house call.*

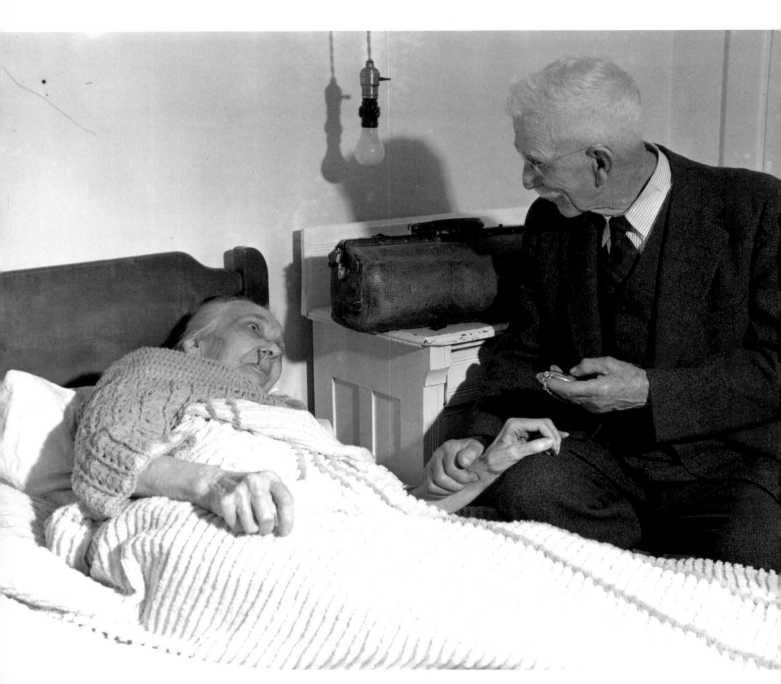

An elderly patient is seen in her bed at home. Ridgway takes her pulse while the thermometer records her temperature.

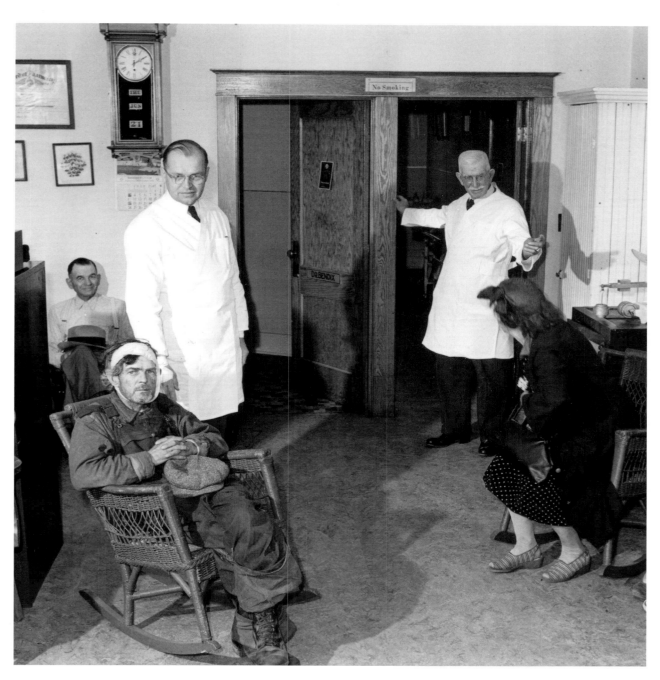

At his clinic in Annandale, Ridgway and an associate invite waiting patients to come back to examining rooms.

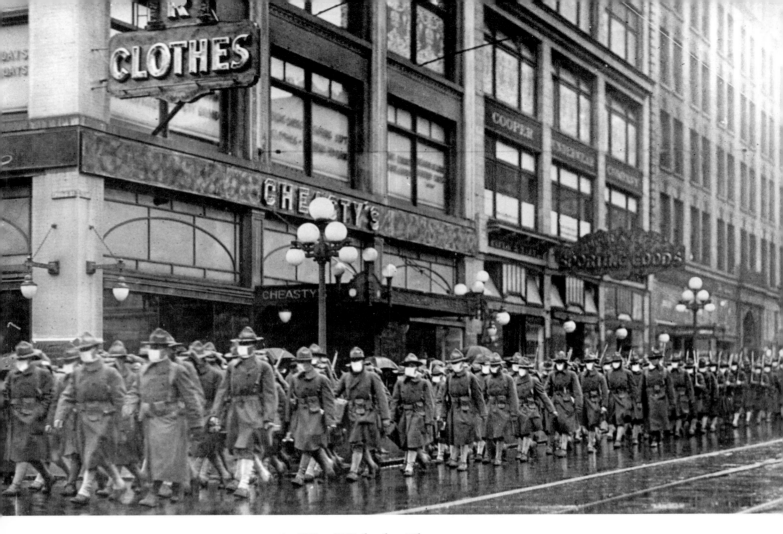

At War With the Flu

In December of 1918, America was in the grip of a major influenza epidemic. The American Red Cross provided masks to these members of the 39th U.S. Army Regiment parading through the streets of Seattle after arriving home from World War I battlefields in France. (American Red Cross.)

Victims of Hookworm

Severe effects of hookworm infection, including extreme anemia and "fisheye" appearance, can be seen in all the members of this Kentucky farm family living in poverty in 1915. (National Library of Medicine, Bethesda, Md. Neg. 67-300)

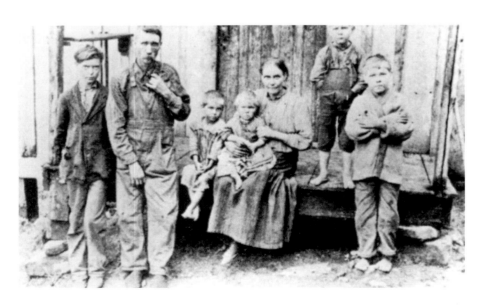

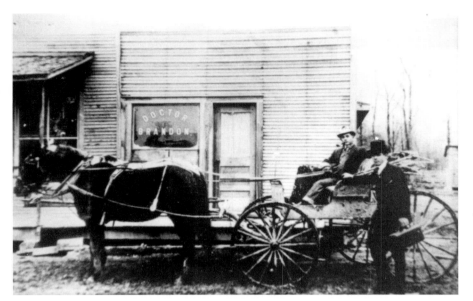

President's Friend
Walter L. Brandon, M.D., stands beside his buggy in front of his office at Broseley, Mo., as he and an assistant prepare to make a house call, circa 1919. He later founded the Brandon Hospital in Poplar Bluff, Mo. Brandon and Capt. Harry S Truman served together in World War I and became lasting friends. (Robert H. Laatsch, M.D.)

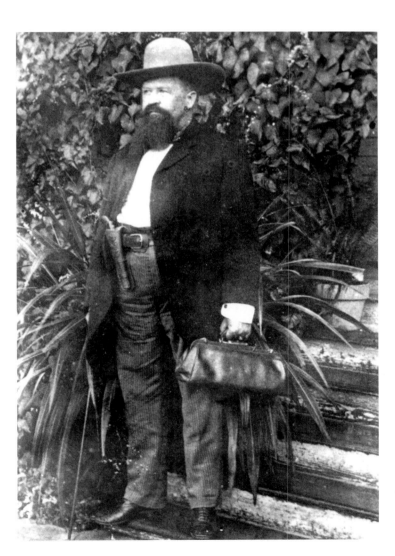

Pistol Packin' Physician
Dr. Hiram Hampton, who practiced medicine in Florida in the early 20th century, usually wore a large pistol on his belt when he traveled the countryside. His wife, Emma, sometimes accompanied him as his nurse. (Florida State Archives.)

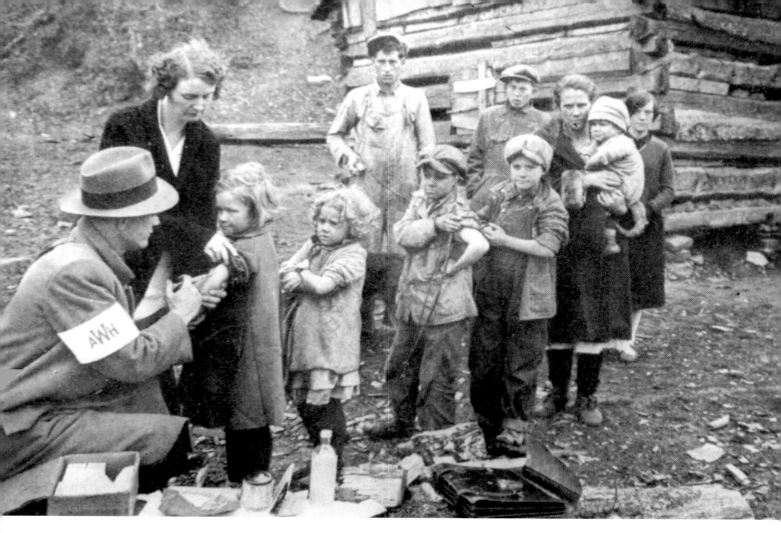

Outdoor Immunization
A physician immunizes mountain children at an outdoor clinic sponsored by the American Women's Hospital Service in 1933 near Spartanburg, S.C. (Archives and Special Collections on Women in Medicine, Allegheny University of the Health Sciences.)

Johnboat Ambulance
When high water blocked roads in eastern Kentucky in 1937, a nurse of the Frontier Nursing Service was assisted by a man and his johnboat in transporting a mother and newborn to the care of physicians at a hospital. The boatsman paddles down a rain-swollen stream with the mother bundled onto a metal cot and the nurse holding the infant. (Frontier Nursing Service, Wendover, Ky.)

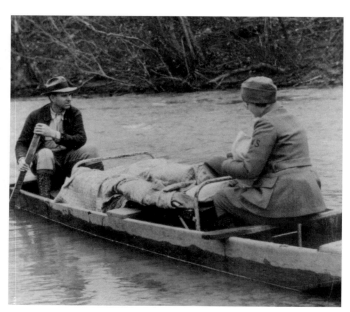

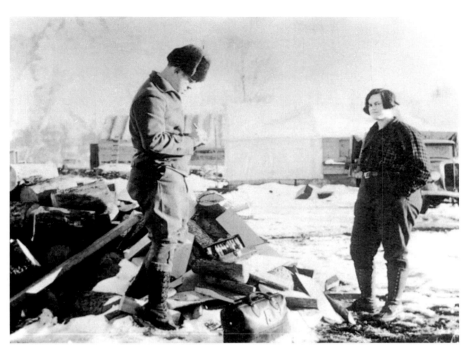

Alaskan Pioneer
C. Earl Albrecht, M.D., writes a prescription for a patient in the 1940s near Palmer, Alaska, where he pioneered health care for a Depression-era farm colony in the remote Matanuska Valley. He directed the military hospital in Anchorage during World War II, and later became Alaska's first full-time health commissioner. Albrecht also helped found the International Union for Circumpolar Health. In 1996, at age 91, he was in ill health and living in Bradenton, Fla. (Margie Albrecht.)

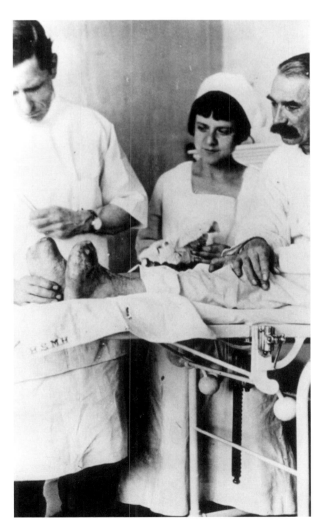

Frozen Feet
Grafton Burke, M.D., working at the Hudson Stuck Memorial Hospital in Ft. Yukon, Alaska, cares for a patient who has lost his toes to frostbite, year unknown. (The Lindberg Collection, Accession number 93-151-390, Archives, Alaska and Polar Regions Department, University of Alaska Fairbanks.)

Care in the Countryside

Lloyd McCaskill, M.D., of the eastern North Carolina farming community of Maxton, cared for the rural people of his region for many years. Bruce Roberts photographed his activities in 1961.

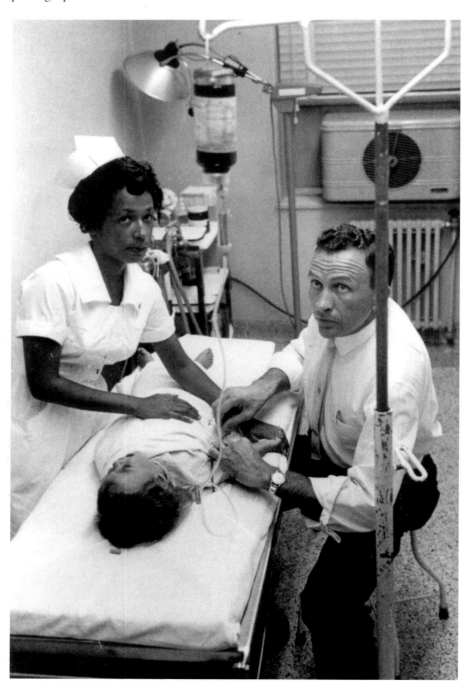

The faces of McCaskill and his nurse reflect their concern as they start an IV drip in a seriously ill child brought to his clinic in Maxton. (Bruce Roberts Photograph Collection, The Center for American History, The University of Texas at Austin. CN08891.)

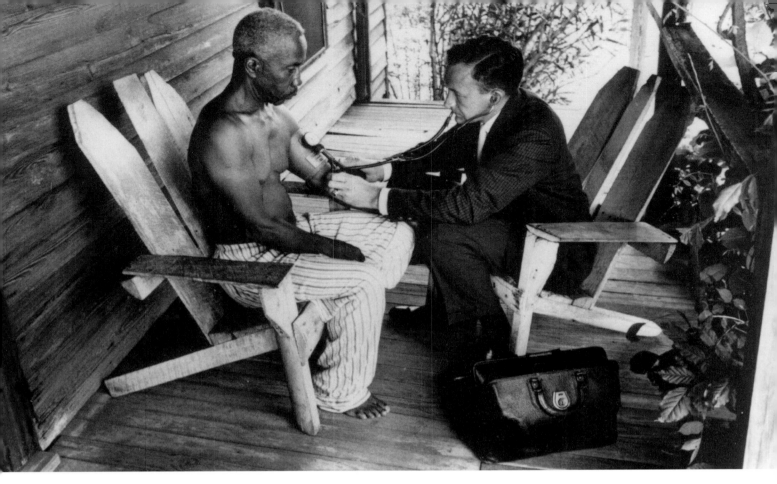

McCaskill takes an elderly man's blood pressure on the front porch of a cabin in an area where cotton and tobacco were the main crops. (Bruce Roberts Photograph Collection, The Center for American History, The University of Texas at Austin. CN08892.)

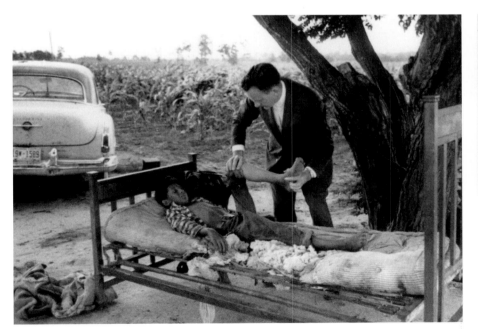

McCaskill was summoned to treat this American Indian boy with a broken leg. The physician examines the injured leg as the boy lies on a ragged mattress in the yard of his farm home. (Bruce Roberts Photograph Collection, The Center for American History, The University of Texas at Austin. CN08705.)

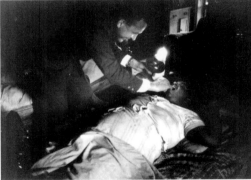

With kerosene lamp in one hand and tongue depressor in the other, McCaskill examines a patient on a late-night house call. (Bruce Roberts Photograph Collection, The Center for American History, The University of Texas at Austin. CN08890.)

45

Medicine in the Mountains

Blaine Cannon, M.D., spent the last 13 years of his life treating rural residents around Balsam Grove, N.C. Trained in leading medical schools and hospitals, he sacrificed to help mountain people desperately in need of medical care. Cannon died of heart disease in 1966 at age 68. Bruce Roberts photographed Cannon.

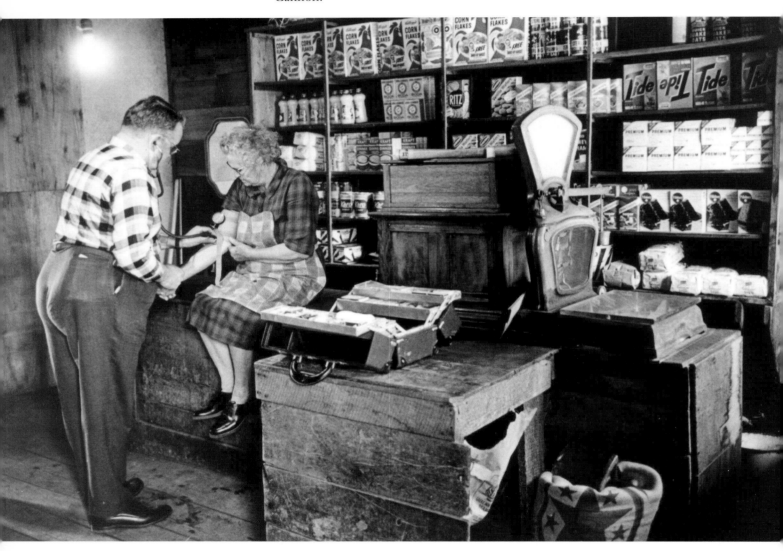

This general store, a 25-mile drive over the mountain from Cannon's clinic in Balsam Grove, is where patients who needed house calls left word for him. After picking up his messages there one day, he checked the blood pressure of the store's proprietress as she sat on the counter. (Bruce Roberts Collection, The Center for American History, The University of Texas at Austin. CN08894.)

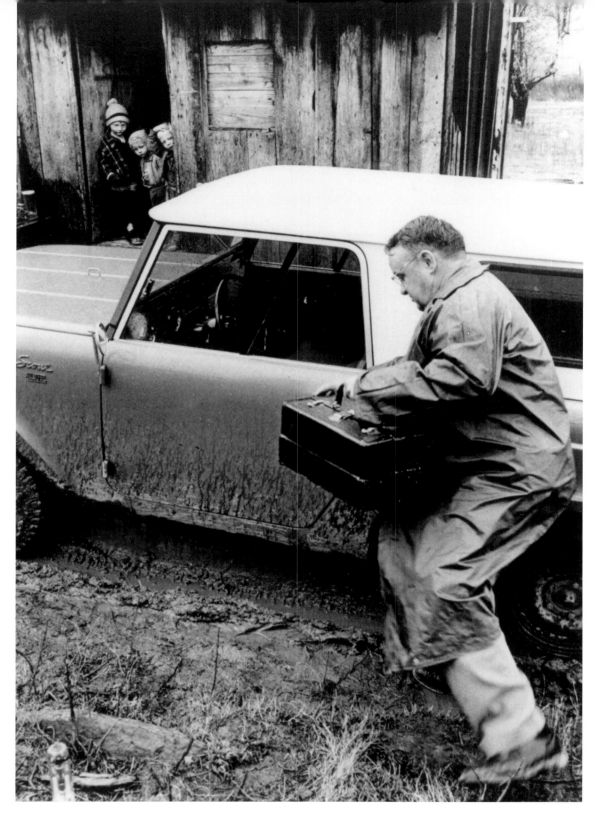

Children wait in the door of their cabin in the Blue Ridge Mountains as Cannon wades mud that challenged his four-wheel-drive International Scout, circa 1960. The children's mother had just borne a baby. Cannon examined the whole family before making his next house call. (Bruce Roberts Collection, The Center for American History, The University of Texas at Austin. CN08895.)

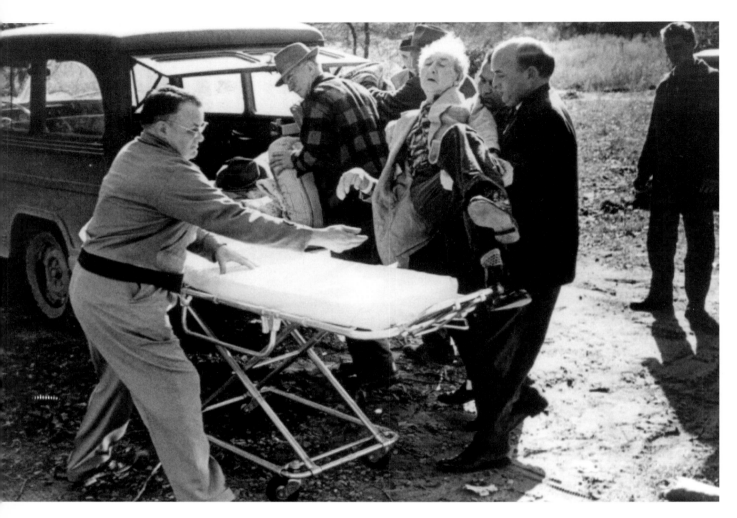

Neighbors transfer Charlie McCall, 75, onto a gurney steadied by Cannon, circa 1958. The physician had found McCall acutely ill in his remote mountain cabin. He loaded the patient into his Jeep station wagon (background), which was fitted with a mattress, and hauled him 15 miles to meet the ambulance at the nearest paved road. (Bruce Roberts Collection, The Center for American History, The University of Texas at Austin. CN08893.)

CHAPTER 3

CARING FOR AMERICA IN 1997

Is there a "typical" family physician? Not really. Family physicians and their practices can differ significantly from one another. The following profiles showcase the personal and practice diversity of today's family physicians.

(Photos by the author.)

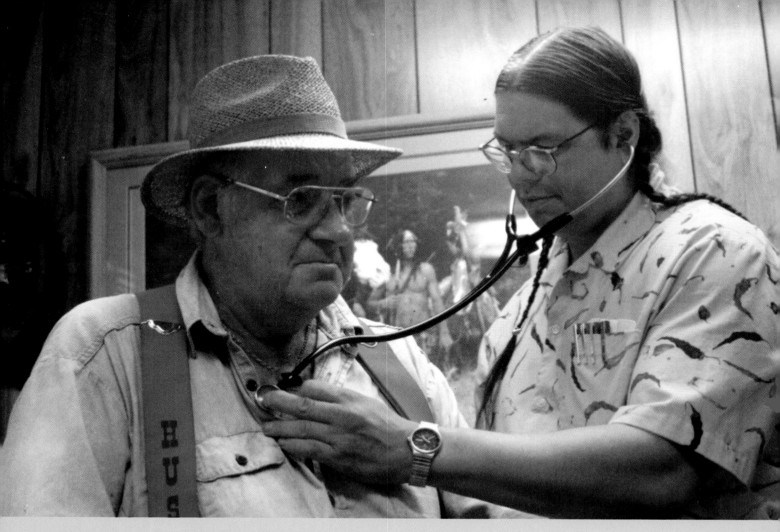

A Mountain Man
Paul Koshney visits Baines for a regular checkup. Koshney, 70 and retired, has spent most of his life working as a millwright and independent logger in the woods of Northwest Idaho. As a young man, he helped build the power plant at the Grand Coulee Dam.

Baines the Teacher
Baines explains an emergency room case to Grant Harbison, left, of Boise, a second-year medical student at the University of Washington who was enrolled in a month-long preceptorship with the physician. Michael Burke, R.N., right, tends to patient Audrey Flowers, Modesto, Calif., whose 84th birthday anniversary dinner was interrupted by an episode of fluid in her lungs.

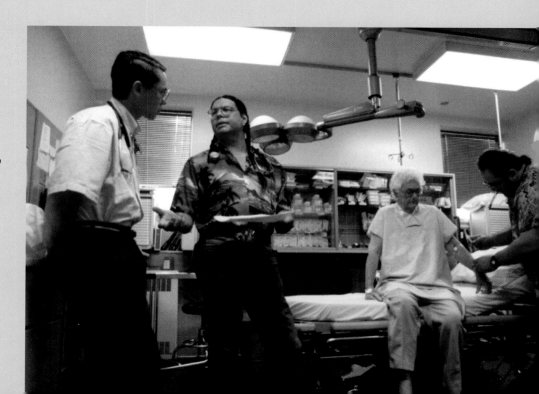

A Maverick Modern Medicine Man

David R. Baines, M.D.
St. Maries, Idaho

*H*is wife nicknamed him Mad Dog. Friends have labeled him the Medicine Man. His patients call him caring and considerate, a physician who displays uncanny insight into their problems and needs.

David Ray Baines, M.D., practices family medicine in the Idaho Panhandle logging community of St. Maries at the edge of the Coeur d'Alene Indian Reservation. Baines, 42, himself a member of the Tlingit and Tsimshian tribes of Southeast Alaska, blends modern medicine with Native American spiritual healing.

The son of a former Methodist minister, Baines now practices traditional Indian religion and incorporates his deep faith in the Creator into his approach to Western medicine. "The power within us comes from the Creator," Baines says of his beliefs. "We are not healers, we are just the enablers to allow the healing spirit to get to the patient. As long as I keep this frame of mind, the healing energy is there for me."

Baines tells of situations where he has melded his traditional medicine, which involves deep spirituality, with his Western medical training.

"One night in Seattle . . . one of the tribal elders came to me in a dream, and I knew she was in trouble," Baines recalls. He sang an Indian song all night—the equivalent of a prayer vigil. "She had been trapped in a car wreck in freezing temperatures. Her body temperature was barely 95 when she was extricated. When I got home and found her at the hospital, she told me she had been calling for me."

Baines also thrives on his participation in medical politics and education. He serves on the clinical faculty of several medical schools and regularly is a preceptor for medical students. His speaking and committee engagements, many on the national level, numbered more than 100 in recent years.

Many of Baines' activities involve his efforts to improve Native American health care. Indians suffer from unusually high rates of obesity, hypertension, diabetes and alcoholism. The tuberculosis rate also is much higher than for the rest of the population.

Four of the major causes of death among Indians—accidents, liver cirrhosis, suicide and homicide—are related to alcohol. There is no evidence that Native Americans are genetically predisposed to alcoholism, although poverty and isolation likely are contributors.

Baines' loyal patients are the benefactors of his training, faith and cross-cultural experience.

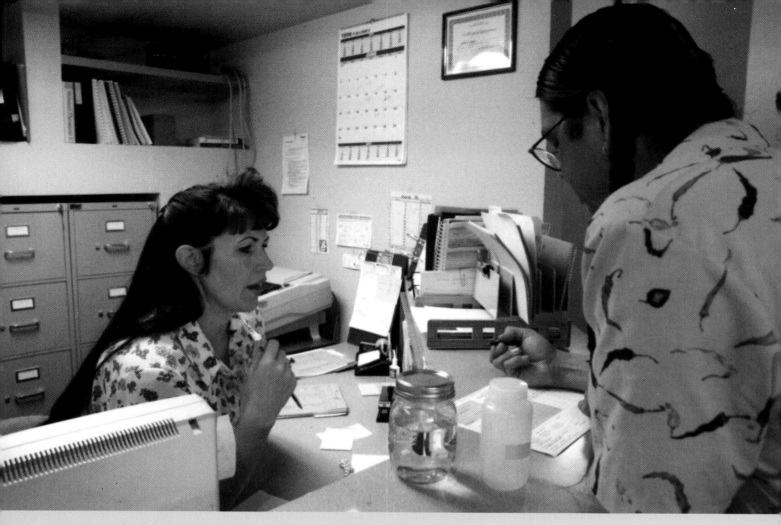

Polluted Water?

Lynda Crane, secretary at the Idaho Department of Health office in St. Maries, accepts a water sample Baines obtained from the Coeur d'Alene River. Residents were concerned about possible lead contamination after flooding disturbed mine tailings.

Paying the Sun's Dues

Baines injects Jack Crane, 66, with a local anesthetic before removing potentially cancerous facial lesions. Crane was exposed to the sun daily for 50 years as a logger and sawmill worker.

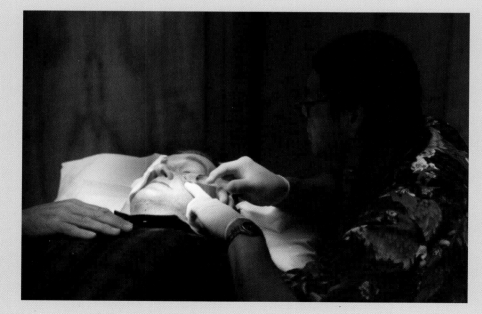

Harry Treloar, an 80-year-old retired boilermaker and millwright, remembers when his family was told he "wasn't going to make it" after suffering a stroke. "Doc Baines stayed with me for three days, and I'm still here," he says. "Any man who can save your life has got to be a good man."

Like most Indian youths growing up on the remote Annette Island Indian Reserve south of Ketchikan, Alaska, Baines expected to earn his living by fishing or logging. Then a freak accident in 1973 drastically changed his life.

Fresh out of high school, Baines was working at the tribal sawmill, clearing a blockage in the huge pipe that carried wood chips to waiting barges. Without warning, the main air compressor kicked on. The explosive blast catapulted the husky 18-year-old 60 feet through the air, slamming him into a dock and crushing both legs.

Fellow workers first thought he was dead. The blast of chips had ripped off most of a new pair of Levis. With his mangled legs bleeding profusely, Baines was hauled in the bed of a pickup to an abandoned airstrip. After long helicopter and ambulance rides, he finally reached a hospital three hours later.

"A pediatrician was going to cast my legs and hope for the best," Baines recalls. "My family intervened, and I was flown to Seattle. I lost 25 pounds and eventually underwent multiple surgeries."

While recuperating from the accident and living with his mother in Phoenix, Baines realized he might never regain full use of his legs. (Two decades later, after sports and riding injuries, his legs now are considered 70 percent disabled.) He began taking classes at a junior college, where a career test indicated a strong aptitude for medicine. He transferred to Arizona State University, soon earned a full scholarship for academic excellence and graduated with honors.

Elated by his acceptance at the prestigious Mayo (Clinic) Medical School in Rochester, Minn., he soon found that the expected stress level was compounded because he was the only Native American there. He cut his long hair in an effort to fit in and avoid hassles from other students. But the loss of his braids made him feel as if he had abandoned his "Indianness." He realized that being an Indian was more important to him than becoming a doctor.

Though his grades were excellent, by the end of his first year he was seriously considering going home to stay. But that summer, he was invited to speak to a group of Native American students in South Dakota. While there, a Sioux medicine man he met during a sacred prayer ceremony in a sweat lodge greatly influenced him. "The medicine man enabled me to have a vision that I should finish school and that I would help people," Baines recalls. That vision was a turning point; he graduated from medical school three years later.

After an internship in Los Angeles and a three-year family practice residency in Cheyenne, Wyo., Baines and his wife, Catherine, a registered dietitian, moved to St. Maries. He soon began helping out at the Indian Health Service clinic on the nearby reservation while building his own private practice in St. Maries. Most of his patients now are white, but he maintains his ties at the reservation clinic.

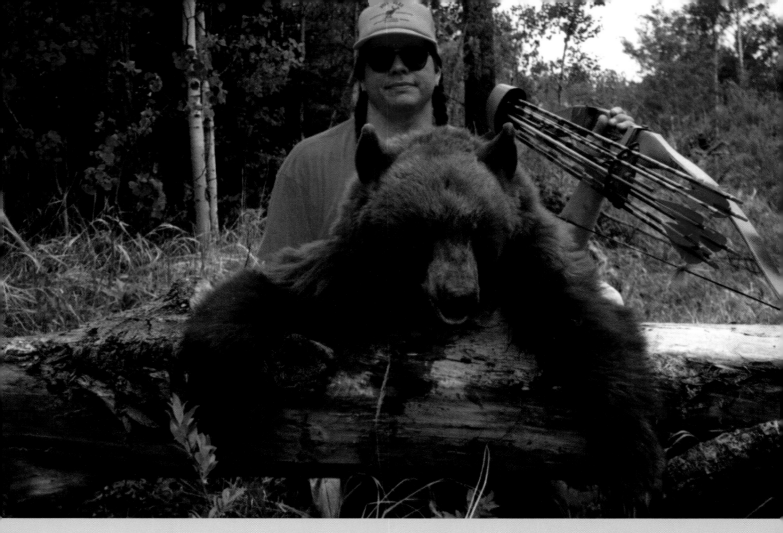

A Spiritual Hunt

A traditional longbow hunter, Baines poses with a prized trophy: a cinnamon-blond phase black bear he killed in 1993 in Saskatchewan after preparing for the hunt with a sacred pipe ceremony. Baines' Tlingit Tribe uses the spirit of the bear as a totem for one of its clans. Some tribes believe killing a bear brings healing powers to the hunter. "I felt that this experience positively influenced me and my practice of medicine," Baines says.

Riding to Relax

Riding his powerful BMW motorcycle, which is adorned with elaborate Native American symbols and his nickname "Mad Dog" (for M.D.), is one of Baines' favorite leisure activities.

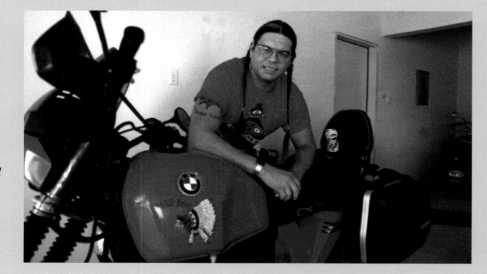

Because of his somewhat maverick lifestyle, Baines also qualifies as one of the few "unorthodocs" in a stereotypical world of coat-and-tie physicians. His long braids, skillfully woven by his wife's nimble fingers, stand out against the bright, custom-tailored shirts that form his office wardrobe. The shirts are sewn by 85-year-old friend Mary McLeod from fabric Baines buys himself.

Ornate Native American theme tattoos, loaded with personal symbolism such as "Better Red Than Dead" and "Mad Dog" (for M.D.), show on each muscular arm when the Medicine Man dons a tight T-shirt and jumps on his bright red BMW motorcycle for a weekend ride. Two-hour basement weight-lifting sessions offer another diversion to relieve the inevitable frustrations of a demanding professional life.

A cherished boon of Baines' existence is the spiritual rejuvenation he enjoys in the sacred sweat lodge of a special friend, Coeur d'Alene medicine man Merle SiJohn. Following ancient native customs, SiJohn carefully crafted the willow-framed lodge at a secluded spot on picturesque Hangman Creek. Baines participates in the medicine man's "sweats" as often as his schedule permits.

An avid outdoorsman and bowhunter since his youth, Baines' living room sports a full-body mount of a 250-pound black bear he took in 1993 in Saskatchewan with one well-aimed arrow from his 75-pound traditional bow. He performed a sacred pipe ceremony showing respect for the bear's spirit before skinning out the animal. Because his tribe uses the bear as the totem of one of its clans, he believes the hunting experience spiritually influenced him and his practice of medicine.

Also in 1993, Baines received the "Gentle Giants of Medicine" award and a $10,000 grant from the Searle pharmaceutical company for his innovative ideas about medicine. He donated the grant to the Association of American Indian Physicians, an organization he formerly chaired, which is dedicated to improving the health of Native Americans.

Although flattered by the award, the laconic Baines says in his characteristic monotone: "I was most excited about the promotion of my respect for all cultures, the spiritual side of medicine and the importance of family medicine as the best way to achieve better health for all Americans."

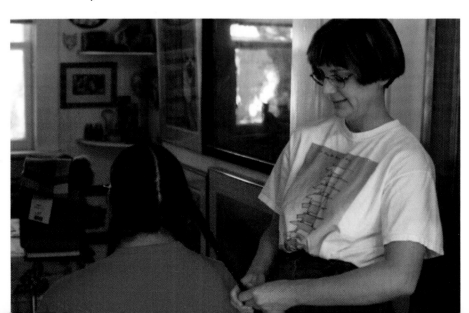

Indian Braids
Catherine Baines braids her husband's hair into traditional Indian pigtails, his normal style.

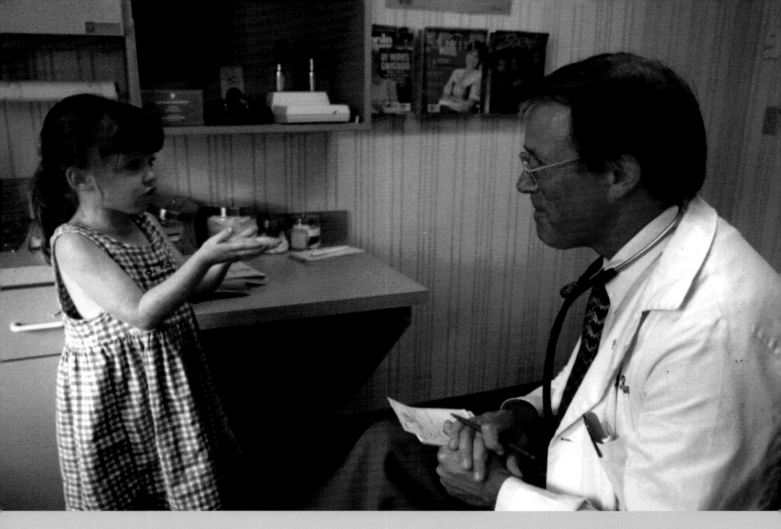

A Patient Listener

4-year-old patient Miranda Walls tells Hartman about a recent experience. Later, she gave him a big hug. Miranda is the daughter of John and Jodie Walls of Kissimmee.

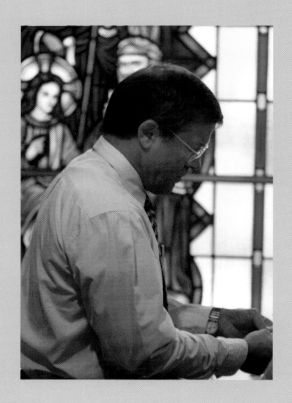

Preparing for the Day

A devout Roman Catholic who considered the priesthood as a young man, Hartman attends morning Mass daily at Holy Redeemer Church in Kissimmee.

A Spiritual Approach to Patients

John R. Hartman, M.D.
Kissimmee, Florida

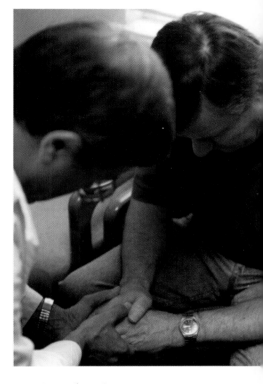

Easing the Concern
Hartman prays with patient Dennis Cable, 49, an operations manager for a chemical company. Cable was concerned about a series of tests he was undergoing for an eye problem.

Anxiety darkens the handsome face of the middle-aged patient as he tells the doctor his worries about an eye problem. Test results so far are normal, but the man still questions why his right pupil is slightly enlarged. He's obviously frightened.

As the doctor keeps talking, the tension eases in the man's face. A mutual sense of trust permeates the tiny room. "May I say a prayer?" the doctor asks, and the patient eagerly grasps his outstretched hands. The two men, both 49, squint their eyes tightly shut. As the healer finishes the brief prayer, the patient's face is calm. Now it will be easier for him to face the results of a CT scan.

John Hartman, M.D., a partner in a small family practice group in Kissimmee, Fla., knows his patients well. He knows what's going on at work. He understands their marital status. He probably can recite the names and ages of their children, who likely are also his patients. And, when a patient is troubled about medical or personal problems, Hartman also knows that nursing the spirit can be part of the healing equation.

A devout Catholic, he enrolled in seminary after high school, thinking he would become a priest. But future wife Cleta Fowler graced his life, and he instead married her and earned an electrical engineering degree from Virginia Polytechnic Institute. But two years into a successful engineering career, he realized that "the fire wasn't there." His deep passion to help his fellow man was much stronger than his desire to continue designing pagers for the Motorola Company.

And so John Hartman began his second career as a student at the University of Miami Medical School. He then completed a family practice residency at the Duke University Medical Center and taught for three years at the Pensacola Naval Air Station Hospital to complete his military obligation. He opened his practice in Kissimmee in 1982.

Why family practice? "For me, there never was any other pathway. I wanted to be a complete physician," says Hartman, who joined the American Academy of Family Physicians immediately on entering medical school. He likely was influenced by his father's career as a medical technologist for the CIA.

"We lived overseas on Saipan and later on Cyprus, and things were a lot more reality-oriented," Hartman recalls. "We had small contingents of people on small islands, and our doctors did everything. My folks often invited these people over to our house and talked about them all the time.

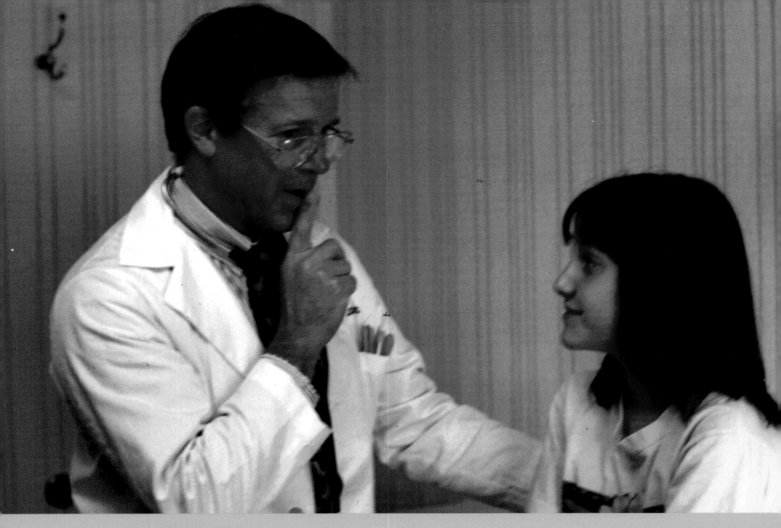

Question From Katie
Katie Nearing, 11, waits for Hartman's answer to a question.
A sixth-grader at Neptune Elementary School, she was there
for a physical prior to attending a summer ecology camp.

"I like family medicine because of the breadth of what can happen. Every day is a little bit different. It's nice to be able to go up to somebody and say, 'I've got a 90 to 95 percent chance of being able to help you. Now, tell me what your problem is.' I get satisfaction out of being able to be the person who meets the needs."

Hartman's patients recite a litany of praise about him.

"I wanted somebody who would take care of everything. I didn't want to get sent back and forth among specialists," says one patient.

"Dr. Hartman sees our whole family as one unit, and that's important," a young mother relates. "It gives us a great feeling of comfort. He always keeps the kids real calm, and they like him a lot. He's honest and never holds anything back from us."

An elderly woman says: "I have many things wrong with me, and he doesn't make me feel like I'm a hypochondriac. Part of my healing process is the time he spends with me. The older you get, the more you need understanding from your doctor. He never hurries, and he makes me feel like I'm a special person."

A teen-ager with a sore throat, accompanied by his father, comes in to see Hartman. The physician obviously is more concerned about the youth's mouth tobacco habit. Hartman addresses the raw throat and then advises the young man that he'll be happy to discuss "what the stakes are" in using snuff, when the teen is ready to listen. "An old proverb says that when the student is ready, the teacher will appear," Hartman tells the grinning youth.

Hartman delivers babies, sets fractures, performs or assists surgeries, counsels patients and makes home visits to shut-ins and the needy. He routinely attends his patients' athletic events, school plays, graduations, weddings and funerals. After he volunteered free care weekly to an increasing homeless population, a fund was started to continue both a clinic and a pharmacy. He also made several trips to the Dominican Republic as part of a medical mission team that worked from dawn to dusk and saw up to 80 patients a day. "Our reward was seeing the thanks they showed in their eyes," the physician recalls.

A Florida rancher's widow tearfully relates how Hartman not only came to their home to be with her husband at his death, but gently comforted and hugged each of her children and other assembled relatives.

He begins most days by attending Mass at Holy Redeemer Catholic Church. After hospital rounds, he reads scripture with his clinic nurse before they begin seeing patients. Seldom preaching, he never imposes his beliefs on others but gently leads them to understand the role he thinks faith plays in good health.

As a high school team physician, Hartman has been a role model for hundreds of athletes and other teens. Some have become family physicians. He also regularly serves as a preceptor who supervises both medical students and family practice residents.

Kissimmee school officials use Hartman as the key physician to discuss "the miracle of the gift of sex" and the "myth of safe sex" with fifth-graders and their parents. He has coordinated church and community efforts at promoting abstinence until marriage.

As a practical businessman as well as a caring physician, Hartman has seen big changes in the practice of medicine. One is "the number of people looking over your shoulder, the insurance companies in particular," he says. "When I began, there really was no case review by the insurance companies. All the bureaucratic red tape with middlemen approving everything and pushing paper makes no sense. I still hospitalize the people who need it, and I don't remember a case where I've not been able to convince the insurance company it's the right thing to do.

"The federal government also can make your life miserable with forms, rules to follow and taxes to pay. But one thing they can't take away from you is the joy of practicing medicine. It's a unique opportunity to help people. I can get a gleam out of the patient's eye at the end of the encounter that is every bit as much payment as the check they write up front before they leave."

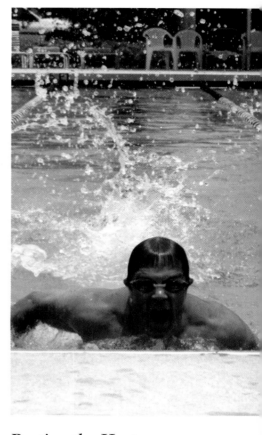

Beating the Heat
Swimming laps at the Kissimmee Aqua Center during his lunch break freshens Hartman for the afternoon. The heat index that June day in steamy Kissimmee was 118.

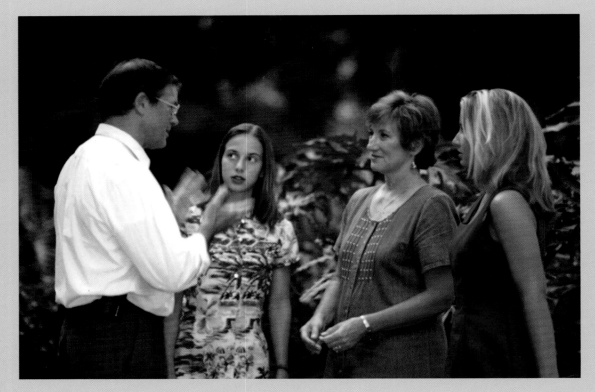

Family Time

Hartman and wife Cleta share time with two of their daughters, high schooler Anne, left, and Heidi, right, a student at Flagler College in St. Augustine. Another daughter, Karen, is an interior designer in Boston.

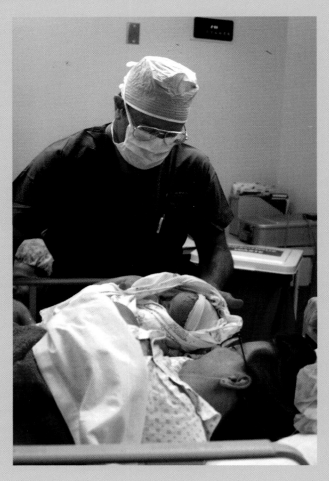

An Introduction

Hartman presents Julie Augsburger, 29, with her first child, 7-pound 15-ounce Kade, minutes after he was delivered by Caesarean section at a Kissimmee hospital. Hartman assisted obstetrician Allan Pratt, M.D., in the delivery. The face of father Bryan Augsburger, who became faint and sat on the floor, can be seen framed under Hartman's right arm.

A Minority Force in Military Medicine

Evelyn Lewis, M.D.
United States Navy

*E*velyn Lewis, M.D., age 41, smashes the fading image of what many Americans used to consider the stereotypical family doctor: white, male, grandfatherly, a graduate of his father's medical school who returned home to Small Town U.S.A. to join Dad's practice. Forget that.

Lewis is a dynamic young African-American who runs five miles and pumps iron every day. She's single and has no children. She turned down an appointment to her father's medical school for fear someone would think he got her in. And she's already practiced medicine and lectured about it from Japan to Haiti to the former Soviet Union.

She's *Commander* Lewis to her colleagues because she proudly wears the whites of a United States naval officer. She teaches at the Uniformed Services University of the Health Sciences in the nation's capital and practices family medicine. Her patients are university students and their dependents.

Lewis grew up in Tampa, Fla. Her mother was a registered nurse. Her parents worked side-by-side in her father's general practice in Tampa. "They opened the clinic at 8 a.m. and locked the door at 1 p.m.," Lewis recalls. "There were no appointments; everyone who signed in got seen. They reopened at 5 and locked up again at 7, usually finishing the last patients about 9:30 at night. My father had a large practice."

Evelyn Lewis was accepted at Nashville's Meharry Medical College, famed as a training ground for black physicians, where her father graduated years earlier. She opted for Brown University's medical school and later transferred to the Chicago Medical School for her last two years of clinical training.

"I knew I wanted to become a doctor from the fourth grade on," says Lewis. She and her brother were "highly encouraged by our parents to do all kinds of things, whatever our interests were." Her brother, an Army medic and senior noncommissioned officer, is nearing 20 years of service in his career.

Lewis wound up in the Navy "because a recruiter happened to be in the right place at the right time." That was the campus cafeteria during her senior year at Spelman College in Atlanta. She later enlisted in the Navy's Health Professional Scholarship Program, which financed her medical training and obligated her to military service.

"I've had an excellent career path, and it's been fun doing it," the ebullient Lewis says as she recalls some of her experiences. After completing her first year of family practice residency at the Jacksonville, Fla., Naval Hospital, she was

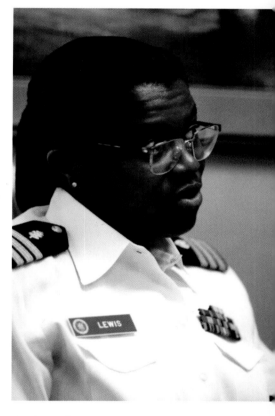

A Good Listener
Lewis listens to a speaker as she sits through one of her many administrative meetings at the Uniformed Services University of the Health Sciences in Bethesda, Md.

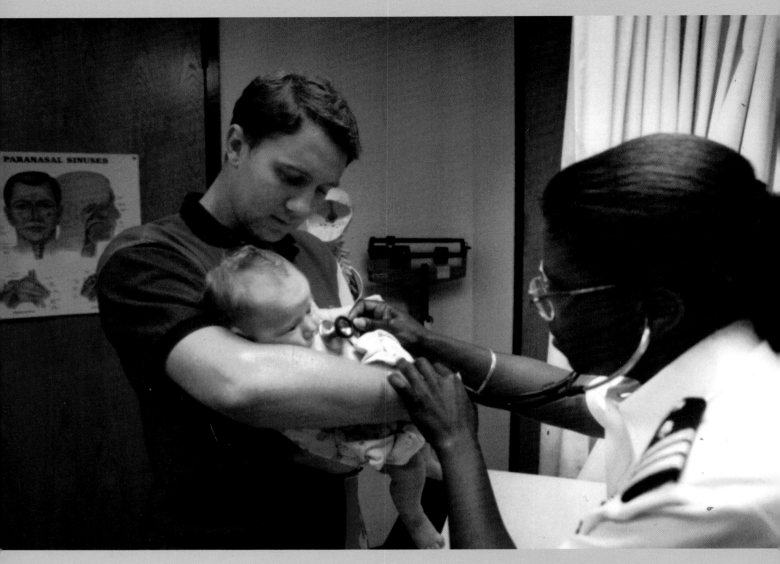

His First Child

Philip Harlow holds his son, Noah, for a checkup seven weeks after his wife, Bernadette, gave birth. Lewis delivered the baby, their first. The mother was a graduate nursing student at the university. Harlow, a former British Army officer, is now a writer.

assigned as the senior medical officer aboard the USS *Simon Lake*, a submarine tender based at Kings Bay, Ga. The ship's crew of 1,500, including 450 females, offered a variety of medical problems for a young physician.

"I treated lots of injuries that needed suturing, and everything else from pregnancy to back pain caused by all the shipboard loading and unloading," Lewis says. "I also saw more serious things like stomach cancer and ulcer disease among the older Navy chiefs, some of whom smoked and drank like there was no tomorrow." She drilled for combat along with the crew, practicing emergency medical procedures while wearing a cumbersome protective suit, helmet and gloves.

After her last two years of residency, she went to Okinawa, Japan, where she opened and ran a clinic for military dependents. There she saw a lot more trauma, including a little boy who was tragically killed when he crashed his bicycle into the side of a car driven by a patient she'd just treated.

While serving as the coordinator of research and behavioral science at the Bremerton, Wash., Naval Hospital in 1992, she got a call from her commanding officer one Friday afternoon. Her assignment: Ship out on Tuesday for Guantanamo Bay, Cuba, to help care for the Haitian refugees who were streaming into the U.S. naval base.

"When I got there, we already had about 15,000 Haitians to take care of," Lewis recalls. "The Navy had turned a restaurant into a clinic and had tents set up outside, one for tuberculosis patients, one for HIV disease, separate ones for kids with measles and whooping cough. There was malaria and lots of parasite problems. We had jars full of huge worms we pulled from patients' mouths and noses."

She was there when the refugees rioted to protest their living conditions. Many of the Haitians and some of the U.S. military personnel were hurt. While she sutured one injured Haitian, the man jerked his head and the needle went through Lewis' finger. "Because most of my patients were from the HIV camp, I remember thinking, 'I hope this one is okay.' I guess I was fortunate. While it was not really a combat zone, it certainly was anxiety-producing," Lewis says.

When the United States began repatriating some of the people back to Haiti, she rode along on a Coast Guard cutter with a pregnant woman. The skipper wouldn't have her on board without a doctor, in case she went into labor.

At her current assignment, Lewis also is heavily involved in minority recruiting at both the faculty and student levels as coordinator of the university's Office of Minority Affairs.

"It's been absolutely wonderful having Commander Lewis here at the university," says Army Lt. Col. Jeannette South-Paul, M.D., chairman of the Department of Family Medicine. "I recruited her because I wanted another clinician who also had good administrative skills, who not only could recruit minorities but also could help with program development. Evelyn Lewis is well-respected throughout the university. Folks recognize her as a high energy person."

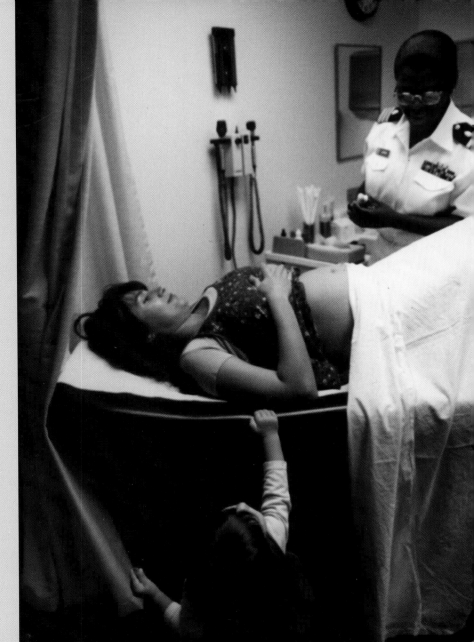

Brother on the Way

Nicola Malakooti, 16 months, reaches up to touch her mother, Susan Malakooti, during a prenatal examination by Lewis at the university's Family Practice Clinic. Malakooti was pregnant with her second child, a boy. Her husband, Mark Malakooti, M.D., a Navy physician, was completing a residency in preventive medicine.

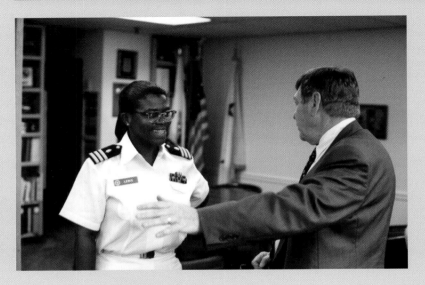

Visiting With President

Lewis drops in for a few minutes of informal conversation with James A. Zimble, M.D., president of the university.

About 15 percent of the university's class of 1997 are minorities, but only 4 percent are black. Asians account for 7 percent and Hispanics 4 percent. South-Paul's goal is to see the percentages climb at least to a proportionate representation of the general population. "People of color bring something special, an understanding and awareness, to the educational environment. We've come quite a ways, and a lot of that is due to the efforts of Evelyn Lewis," South-Paul says.

Citing U.S. military peacekeeping and humanitarian involvement in the Middle East, Haiti, Bosnia and Somalia in recent years, South-Paul sees a great need for diversity among armed forces leaders and physicians. "Military doctors are increasingly exposed to people who are not traditional, white, middle-Americans. We're seeing multicultural people with different values and speaking different languages, not just overseas but right here in this country. Our faculty and students need to look more like the people we serve."

Evelyn Lewis is doing her part to accomplish that mission. She's also promoting careers in family practice, a key military medicine specialty. More than 20 percent of the recent graduates at the university have entered family practice residencies. Thanks to another Lewis initiative, the university now has a highly successful mentoring program that links each student to a faculty member. Helping students overcome obstacles is what Lewis enjoys most about her job. And they'd be amused by her understatement when she says, "I'm an advocate for them."

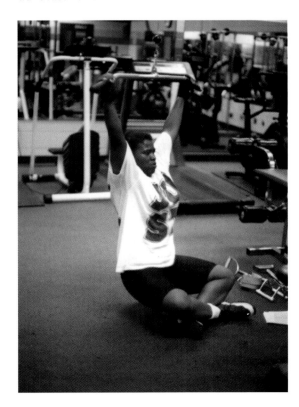

Keeping Fit
Lewis works out regularly in the university's gym to stay in shape and meet the Navy's physical fitness requirements.

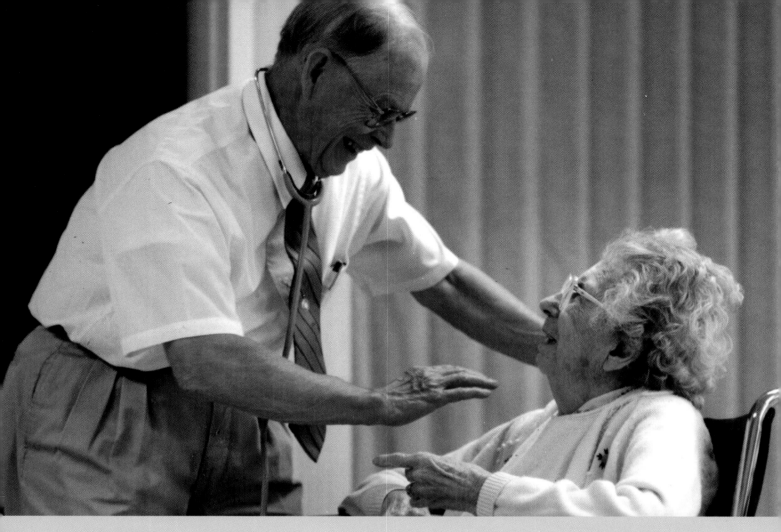

Old Friends

Macdonnell reminisces with longtime friend Earlie George as he makes rounds at a Marshfield nursing home.

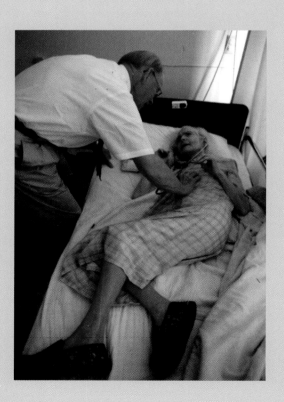

70 Years of Macdonnell Care

Iva Francis, now 102 years old, was Macdonnell's boyhood Sunday school teacher at the First Baptist Church in Marshfield. He gives her a checkup at a nursing home. His father, C.R. Macdonnell, M.D., was Francis' physician from 1928 until his death in 1966, when "Dr. Tommy" assumed her care.

A Medical Legacy in Missouri's Hills

Tommy Macdonnell, M.D.
Marshfield, Missouri

"Don't bother with him, he's not going to make it anyway," the combat medic said after his partner dropped the end of Tommy Macdonnell's stretcher. Macdonnell remembers he relaxed, put himself "totally in God's hands" and then lost consciousness.

The 22-year-old sergeant woke up three weeks later in a hospital in France with a fractured skull, vision and hearing loss, broken ribs and multiple shrapnel wounds. The same land mine had killed the young soldier fighting beside him on that frigid day in January of 1945 during the Battle of the Bulge.

Fortunately for Macdonnell and the thousands of people whose lives he would touch later, his World War II experiences convinced him to return home and become a family doctor like his father and grandfather.

"I was fed up with all the killing. I wanted to begin saving lives and help humanity in a different way," Macdonnell recalls. A half-century later, the semiretired physician known as "Doctor Tommy" to thousands of patients and friends has become a living legend in his home region of Southwest Missouri.

Macdonnell, now 74, saw his first combat on D-Day in the famed Normandy Invasion. Bleeding from a hip wound, he rolled into the filth of a German latrine and crawled within 150 yards of an enemy bunker. He used the shooting skill he learned from his father to put the first round from his M-1 rifle through a German observation scope. That bullet silenced enemy artillery and mortars in the area. And it earned Macdonnell the Silver Star Medal, America's second-highest award for heroism. Wounded again later that day, he spent months in a British hospital before being sent back to battle.

Macdonnell returned home after the war and earned a bachelor's degree in medicine from the University of Missouri–Columbia. He was accepted at Indiana University's school of medicine. A job as a clinic janitor paid for his room. Army disability benefits provided tuition, food and other expenses.

"During my clinical training, I fell in love with every specialty," Macdonnell recalls. Working extra time in an obstetrics program as a senior, he once made 30 home deliveries in two weeks, including four in one night in different homes. After graduation, Macdonnell developed and completed a two-year residency in general practice, one of the earliest in the country, at Kansas City, Mo., General Hospital. His thorough training in obstetrics and pediatrics had prepared him well to join his father's practice in Marshfield, Mo., in 1952. He brought along his new wife, Ann Martin Macdonnell, a nurse he'd met in Indianapolis.

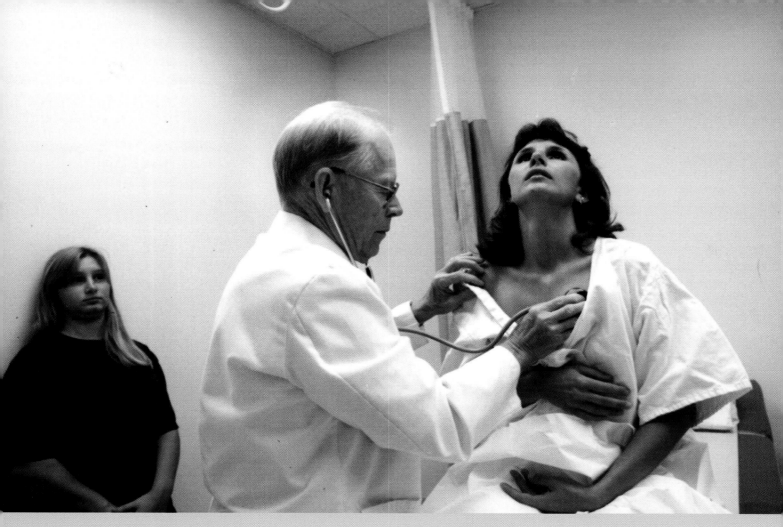

Learning From Mom

Florence Bradley, 38, is examined by Macdonnell during a Well-Women's Clinic at the Webster County Health Unit. The health unit, which moved into a new building in 1996, was founded by Macdonnell's father, C.R. Macdonnell, M.D., in 1957. Bradley brought along her daughter, Jennifer, 14, left, so she would know what to expect at her own examination, scheduled for several days later.

Well-Women's Clinic

Marguaret Pettitt, 45, jokes with nurse practitioner Marilyn Trumble as Pettitt undergoes a pelvic examination by Macdonnell at the county health unit. When Pettitt was 12 years old, she inhaled a brass straight pin and underwent lung surgery by Macdonnell's father.

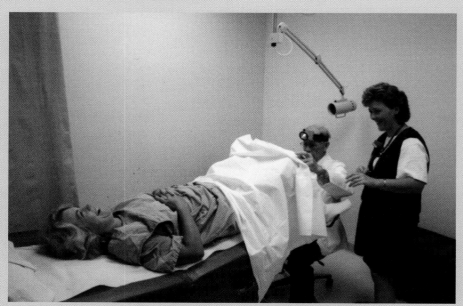

C.R. Macdonnell had practiced in Marshfield, a county seat town in the Ozark Mountains, since 1928. Patients still insisted on seeing him. The receptionist asked a patient one day: "Did you come to see Tommy or the Doctor?" The senior Macdonnell stepped out of his office and announced: "It's Doctor Tommy. He has his M.D. degree." From then on, they were "Dr. C.R." and "Dr. Tommy."

Still, the young doctor was not in great demand. "Daddy would have a waiting room full of folks, and I'd be twiddling my thumbs," Dr. Tommy recalls. "So he sent me out on house calls. Patients eventually accepted me."

In 1953, the Macdonnells left their office on the town square and built a modern clinic at the edge of town. The clinic had private rooms for new mothers, eight examining rooms, a fracture room and an ambulance entrance. They saw plenty of trauma cases from the heavy traffic whizzing by the clinic on legendary U.S. Route 66. The nearest hospital was 25 miles away at Springfield.

Dr. C.R. died in 1966, but not before he had delivered six of Tommy and Ann's eight children. Dr. Tommy, who idolized his father, attended each birth. "Daddy knew things about obstetrics that even doctors today haven't learned. He was a learned man and a wonderful physician," Macdonnell recalls, his voice trailing off.

In carrying on the tradition, Tommy Macdonnell presided over 4,582 deliveries before heart surgery slowed him down in 1983. "That's not counting lots of twins and several sets of triplets," he says. In more than a dozen cases, he drove over snow-covered hill roads in a four-wheel-drive truck to reach mothers in labor.

A 1989 medical book featured a photograph of Macdonnell with about 200 of his grown "babies" on the courthouse lawn.

"My first delivery in Marshfield was a young woman I'd never seen," Macdonnell says. "Her mother called and said the daughter 'had a misery in her body.' That's an old Ozarks term meaning she was in labor. I grabbed my OB bag, drove to the home and told the woman she was going to have twins, one head first and the other feet first.

"The grandmother moaned and said she'd seen that once and the doctor had broken a baby's neck. She didn't remember the doctor's name, but said he was traveling with a (medicine) show going through town. Anyway, I delivered two healthy boys and didn't break a neck. I charged $25, which they never paid. One boy grew up to be a store manager, and the other one ended up in prison."

After his heart surgery, Macdonnell sold the large clinic and built a smaller one. Always interested in government, he ran for the Missouri House of Representatives in 1985 as a Democrat. He handily defeated his opponent in a heavily Republican district. His campaign slogan was: "We need a doctor in the House." Friends teased that he literally had "delivered" enough votes to win.

Besides his legislative duties, the only doctor in the House also ran a free clinic out of his Capitol office and took care of some 300 legislators and staffers. He dispensed samples supplied by drug companies.

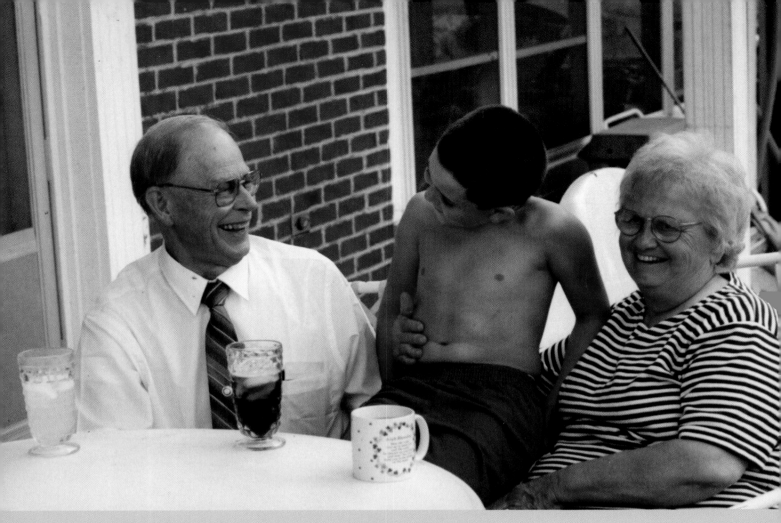

Happy Grandparents

Ann Macdonnell and her husband enjoy grandson Cole Alexander, 10, who lives next door. The genial and unflappable mother of eight laughs when she remembers former Missouri Gov. Joe Teasdale stopping at their home while campaigning. "He needed to wash and change shirts before attending a political rally in Marshfield," she recalls. "I was mortified later to discover the wash cloth I'd given the governor had a big hole in it."

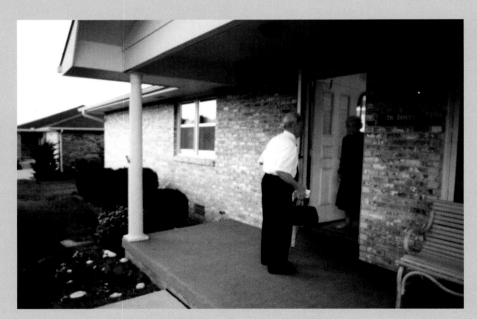

An Evening House Call

Helen Roper greets Macdonnell at her front door as he arrives to check on swelling in her legs. He already has put in a 12-hour day before making the house call near dusk. The physician and patient are lifelong friends.

Macdonnell's legislative successes included smoke-free public buildings, required student immunizations, a teen smoking law, an Office of Rural Health, nurse practitioner programs, Medicaid revisions and stricter licensing for residential care facilities.

Macdonnell also found time to serve on the local school board and two college trustee boards and to fulfill dozens of other civic and professional obligations. Service awards crowd the walls of his modest home office.

He retired from the legislature at the end of 1994 and sold his Marshfield clinic, which he had continued to operate with a partner. By that time, Macdonnell had amassed medical charts on some 20,000 patients.

His "retirement" lasted only two days. On Jan. 4, 1995, he began a half-time job with the Missouri Department of Health, overseeing maternal and family health in a 21-county area. After repeat heart surgery a year later, he was back on the job in less than two months.

These days, a tireless Tommy Macdonnell still conducts women's and children's clinics for several county health departments. He makes house calls and nursing home visits in Marshfield and takes care of elderly patients. Some, like his 102-year-old former First Baptist Church Sunday school teacher, were among those who insisted on seeing only his father 45 years ago.

The Macdonnells' comfortable country home bustles with the coming and going of children and grandchildren every day. And he has more time to tend his prize bull, Charley, and the small herd of beef cattle that roam the Macdonnells' 255-acre home place on the outskirts of Marshfield.

To know Dr. Tommy Macdonnell is to understand his deep love for his fellow man. To witness the high esteem in which he is held by his patients is to appreciate the 70-year legacy of Macdonnell medical care.

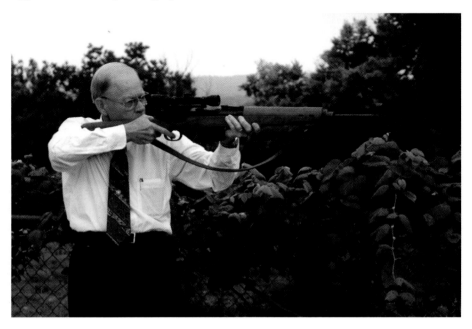

A Personal Souvenir

Macdonnell, a highly decorated combat veteran of World War II, shows off a sniper rifle that nearly killed him. Alerted by fleeing deer, Macdonnell dropped to the ground just as the Nazi sniper's bullets whizzed over his head. He stealthily circled the wooded area, surprised and captured the enemy rifleman and brought the weapon home. Macdonnell, a lifelong hunter and marksman, enjoys shooting the German rifle occasionally.

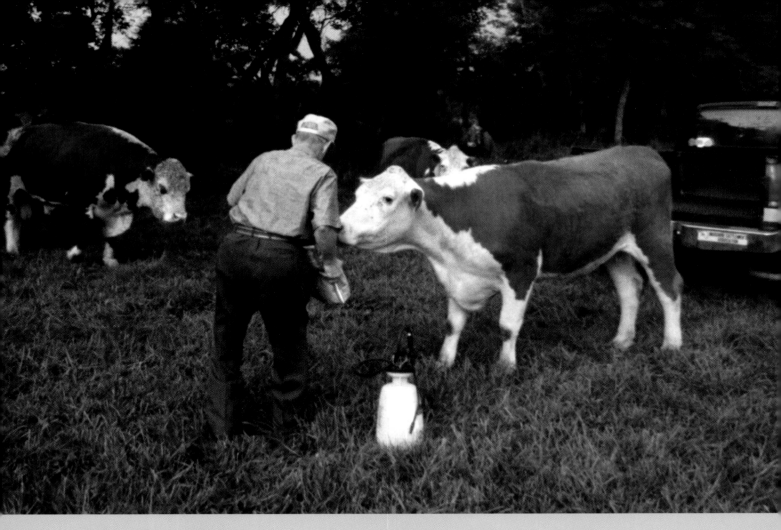

Here Comes Charley

Attracted by the feed he's scattering, a curious cow noses Macdonnell as prize bull Charley approaches from left. Macdonnell has enjoyed raising beef cattle as a diversion from the stresses of practicing medicine.

Politicking

Macdonnell attends a campaign reception in nearby Springfield, Mo., for State Rep. Craig Hosmer, left, a family friend who grew up on a farm near Macdonnell's home. Others are Missouri House Speaker Steve Gaw and Jim Blaine, M.D., right, a family physician and president of the Greene County Medical Society. Macdonnell, a Democrat, served four terms as a state representative in a heavily Republican district.

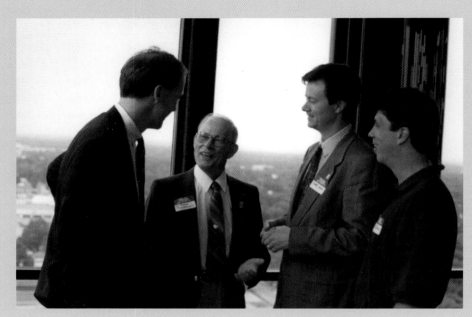

A Model Physician for Managed Care

Leland L. Fairbanks, M.D.
Mesa, Arizona

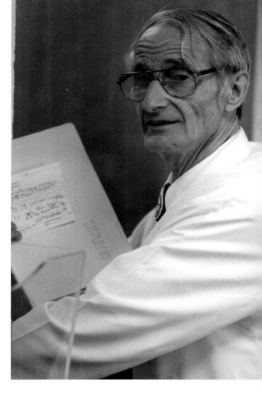

ew patients of Leland Fairbanks, M.D., 67, know that their kindly, unassuming family physician has quietly crusaded for humanitarian causes around the world for more than four decades.

His mild manner and deceptively wispy countenance belie an inner passion that drives him not only to heal his patients but also to try to cure the social ills around him.

Fairbanks retired in 1988 from a 30-year career with the U.S. Public Health Service. He devoted most of that tenure to the Indian Health Service, twice taking time out for two-year tours of duty in Liberia. He now works for a health maintenance organization (HMO), seeing from 20 to 30 patients daily at CIGNA Healthplan's Stapley Health Care Center in Mesa, Ariz.

Recognized internationally as a pioneer in fighting the health risks of tobacco, Fairbanks has represented the United States 11 times at international symposiums, including the World Conference on Tobacco and Health this year in Beijing, China. As president of Arizonans Concerned About Smoking, he helped spearhead the 1996 ballot vote that banned smoking in Mesa's public places. And, he was a primary catalyst in making Public Health Service facilities smoke-free.

Fellow tobacco warrior Ann Robb, M.D., a family physician who practices in nearby Tempe, credits Fairbanks' anti-tobacco efforts with "saving more lives than all the heart surgeons combined. He's also the most savvy, decent, humble, honest and effective family physician I know. I consider him a wonderful role model and mentor."

Born in southeastern Minnesota in 1930, during America's Great Depression, Fairbanks attended eight different schools while his father sought work as a laborer. His parents had lost their family farm when fire destroyed the barn and they couldn't meet mortgage payments. Those firsthand experiences taught a young Lee Fairbanks what being needy meant and sowed the seeds of his humanitarian interests.

He graduated with honors from Augsburg College in Minneapolis, where he loaded freight trucks at night to pay expenses. After he married sweetheart Eunice Picha, a Minnesota farm girl, she helped him make his way through the University of Minnesota Medical School. That's where he first got to know a black person, a medical student from Nigeria who was about to flunk out because he couldn't master the American testing system.

Only Fairbanks showed up to testify at a hearing where the Nigerian was given a second chance. Other students stayed away because they feared being

On the Move
Fairbanks pauses momentarily at the door of an exam room to listen to a nurse's question. At age 67, the energetic physician is well into a second career after retiring with 30 years of service from the Public Health Service.

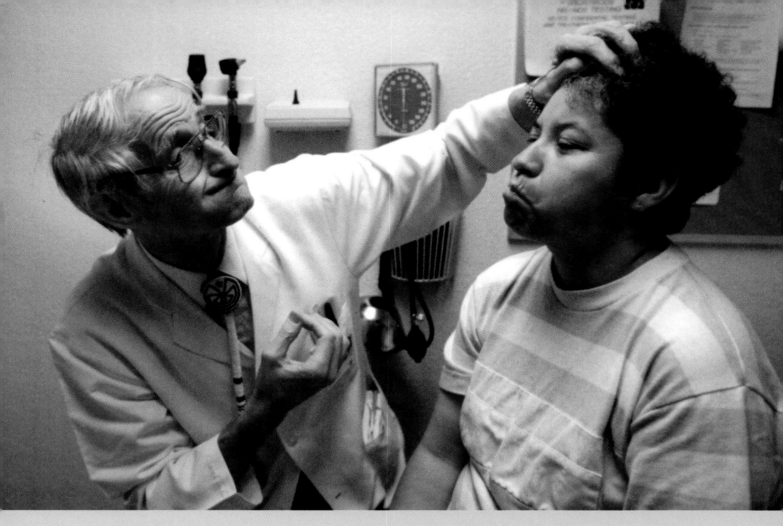

A Medical Mimic

*Fairbanks mimics Antonia Robledo, a Bell's palsy patient in for a follow-up exam.
He's elated with the progress she's made in regaining facial functions.*

Skin Cancer Concern

*Fairbanks shows Irene Sainz,
36, an auto dealership
employee, photos of potentially
cancerous skin lesions. She has
come in to let him examine a
mole on her back.*

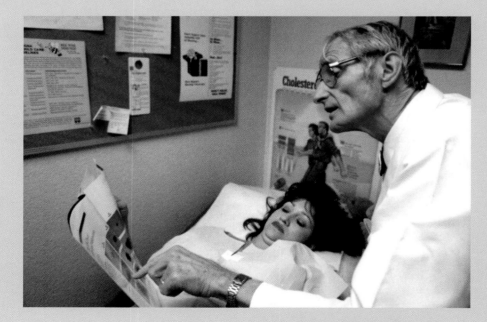

branded as troublemakers if they spoke up for the African. The Nigerian earned his medical degree and became a physician in his native land.

"We've always tried to support people being treated equally without regard to whether they are male or female or what the color of their skin is. We never did a whole lot of marching. We just stood for what we thought was right," Fairbanks says with a quiet intensity.

While working as a young intern in New Orleans in 1958, Fairbanks encountered Deep South racial attitudes. En route to work each morning, he sat in the back of the bus with the "coloreds." His support helped give them the courage to gradually move to the front and finally integrate the transit system. The 3,500-bed Charity Hospital of Louisiana, where he worked, had separate elevators for blacks and whites. While rushing a bottle of blood to an emergency transfusion one day, Fairbanks boarded the black elevator because it was much closer to his destination on another floor. Word quickly spread. Within a week, employees of both races were riding the most convenient elevators, and the custom quietly ended.

Two years later, while completing a family practice residency in Norfolk, Va., Fairbanks protested the closure of the public schools in Prince George County because of desegregation. When white Methodists vacated their church in a "transitional" neighborhood and invited the Fairbanks family to come along to a suburban location, they refused. Instead, they became the only white members of the otherwise-black Methodist congregation that occupied the old building.

In 1962, Fairbanks took his wife and two small children to Liberia for two years. He was chief physician for the U.S. Peace Corps volunteers in that West African country. Later, he moved his young family back to Liberia and spent two more years at the John F. Kennedy Memorial Medical Center in the capital city of Monrovia. There, he directed the training of Liberian nurses, midwives and physicians. He also practiced clinical family medicine and cared for both pediatric and obstetric patients at a maternity hospital.

"We had some frightening experiences living in Africa with two small children," Eunice Fairbanks recalls. "We had a couple of break-ins at our home. Once, I woke up to see a man crawling into our bedroom on the floor. He had climbed through the bars on our windows. I screamed, and he ran away. Most of the crime was petty thievery, and nobody got hurt. Sometimes if a thief got caught out in the villages, they would cut off his hand."

Another African experience fueled Fairbanks' fervor to fight tobacco. That was his discovery that Liberia and other needy nations were forced to accept U.S. tobacco if they were to receive American food aid.

"I was troubled that we were taking advantage of these poor people who had not been educated about tobacco's dangers," Fairbanks recalls.

Though his patients know little of this modest man's background, they quickly discover his skills and sincerity.

"His compassion sets him apart from other physicians," says office nurse

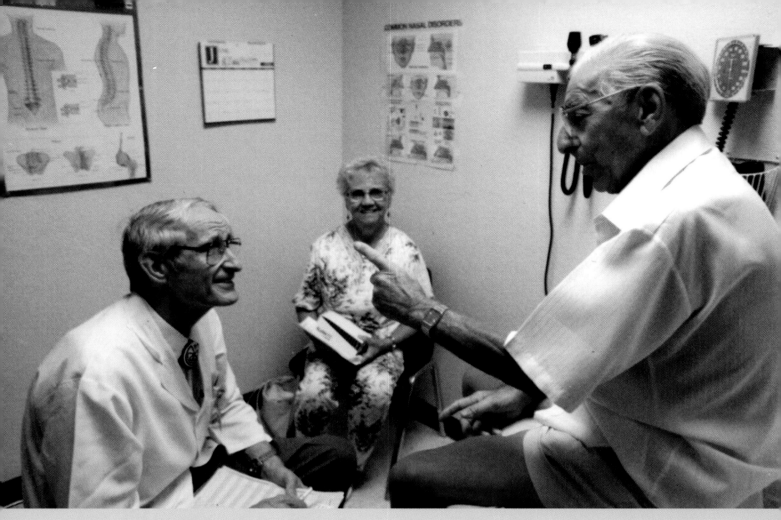

Chester's Sales Pitch

Chester Galluzzo, who has multiple health problems, describes one of them to Fairbanks as Geraldine Galluzzo, his wife of 55 years, watches. Galluzzo, a retired auto sales manager, came in for an exam one day before his 82nd birthday anniversary.

Anti-Smoking Guns

Huddling during a Mesa City Council meeting, Fairbanks and his friend, Stan Turley, talk strategy. Veteran politician Turley formerly was president of the Arizona Senate and speaker of the Arizona House. In the 1970s, he introduced Arizona's first anti-tobacco legislation, which curtailed smoking in elevators. Turley and Fairbanks supported Proposition 200 in 1996, which banned smoking in public places in Mesa.

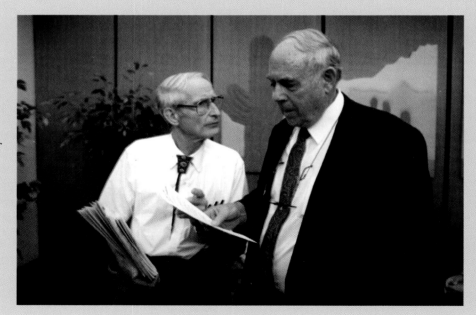

Mary Ann Epp, who has worked with Fairbanks for years. "Sometimes, older people come in, and their eyes start swelling with tears. They really don't need a physician, just somebody to talk to about their problems. He's the one who will listen. He won't rush them out at the end of their 15-minute appointment."

Geraldine Galluzzo, whose husband, Chester, has multiple health problems, says, "We've never had a doctor who is so attentive to us or so punctual when there are test results we need to know about."

"He'll pick up the phone at 9 o'clock at night and let us know about my lab reports," says Chester Galluzzo, age 82. "You'd never know he's been working all day and is probably really tired."

Fairbanks also spends time on the phone consulting subspecialists "if I need their advice," he says. "HMOs sometimes are criticized for avoiding referrals just to save money, but I don't do that. And, if a patient is not comfortable without seeing a subspecialist, then I refer them."

He gives CIGNA, his employer, "really high marks for their medical records system and clerical support. When I have a patient on the phone and need a chart, they get it to me in a hurry. That really helps." Fairbanks sees properly managed HMOs as a key to providing good health care while containing costs.

Retired Phoenix-area oncologist Clifford Harris, M.D., a principal founder of CIGNA, encouraged Fairbanks to go to work for the HMO. "Lee Fairbanks is exactly the type of family physician HMOs need," Harris says. "He's totally committed to his patients."

"The best way to improve medical costs is better prevention and better care," Harris says. He cites the many studies his HMO has done to standardize and improve treatment protocols, drastically reducing hospital stays and saving millions of dollars.

"In a managed care situation, you worry about the whole patient population. You can really make a difference in the quality and cost of health care," Harris says.

Leland Fairbanks often makes a difference simply with a "prescription" of information and advice on how patients can help themselves. Because they trust him and follow his suggestions, patients often recover without needing expensive drugs. He also has been known to reach into his billfold and loan money voluntarily to an elderly patient who needed medication immediately but had left her purse at home.

Providing as much information as possible to each patient is one of Fairbanks' highest priorities. He faithfully returns calls and reports all available lab results to patients before leaving his desk at the end of his typical 10- to 12-hour days.

His patients don't care if he's late for their appointments, nurse Epp says. "They know that when they get in that exam room, he'll take all the time needed to take care of their problem."

As they enjoy the sunset years of her husband's medical practice in Arizona, Eunice Fairbanks declares, "We're happier now than we've ever been." You can be sure they aren't any happier than the patients fortunate enough to have Lee Fairbanks for their family physician.

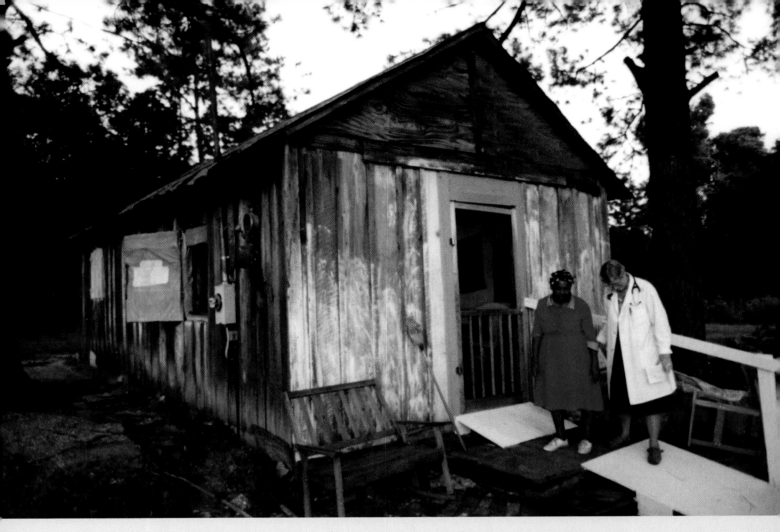

Country House Call
Sister Roseanne Cook talks to Willie Reeds on the front porch of the small home Reeds shares with cancer patient Jesse Morrisette, about 10 miles from Cook's clinic. Their only water is a faucet in the front yard.

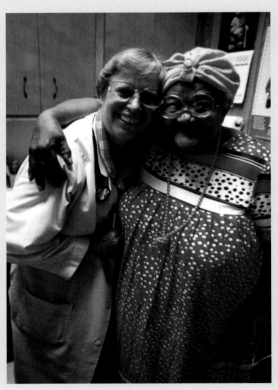

'A Sweet Doctor'
Patient Margaret Lymon, 75, gives Sister Roseanne a playful hug after her examination at the clinic in Pine Apple, Ala. "She's a sweet doctor and she's my standby," Lymon says lovingly of Sister Roseanne.

Dedicated to Serve in Rural Alabama

Sister Roseanne Cook, M.D.
Wilcox County, Alabama

Against the drone of insects in the sweltering South Alabama afternoon, bedfast Jesse Morrisette hears the vehicle slow down and pull off the blacktop into the front yard of the tiny cabin. His common-law wife, Willie Reeds, calmly greets their visitor, who walks through the front door with a smile on her face.

Morrisette, 75, manages a wan smile in return as he sits up in bed with the help of his guest. The visitor is Sister Roseanne Mary Cook, M.D., 58, one of the bright spots in their simple lives. Sister Roseanne is a member of the Sisters of St. Joseph of Carondelet, a Roman Catholic order. She's also a family physician making a house call. There's little she can do now for Morrisette except make him comfortable. That's all he expects. He's slowly dying of esophageal cancer. His mate cares for him in the one room they occupy in their board-and-batten home.

The cabin has no plumbing, but Reeds proudly confirms that they now have water—a faucet in the front yard. A bare light bulb in a porcelain ceiling fixture illuminates the room. Wallpaper chickens march single-file around a border below the ceiling. The white walls are hung with five large tapestries bearing stags, lions and other wild animals.

Morrisette lies atop a red bedspread in the breeze of a large floor fan that fights the stifling heat that's intensified by a wood-fired cookstove. His pillow cases match the blue and white quilt on the foot of the bed in the corner of the neat room.

Reeds rocks behind the stove while Sister Roseanne grasps her patient's hands and talks to him. Then the doctor invites Reeds outside for a solemn conversation that ends in a hug. Now they both know that Morrisette probably won't leave the house again until the undertaker comes. (That happened several weeks later.)

"When we know there's no other treatment that can change their disease and it's terminal, if they want to stay at home I make every effort to make them comfortable there. I arrange for an IV morphine drip or injections for pain through a home health service. It's better for both the family and the patient," Sister Roseanne says.

She has dedicated her life to caring for the residents of Wilcox County, 50 miles southwest of Montgomery. Morrisette was typical of many of her 2,500 patients. He could sign his name only with an "X." He was old, poor and black. He lived 25 miles from the nearest hospital.

Roseanne Cook was a 20-year-old college sophomore with a boyfriend

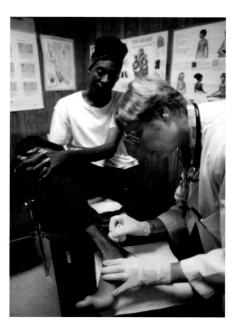

Sickle Cell Patient
Sister Roseanne Cook dresses the ankle ulcers of Erick Blackmon, 18, a victim of sickle cell disease. Blackmon has been hospitalized several times and periodically gets blood transfusions to enhance healing. The disease affects about 50,000 Americans, most of them black. Many patients are crippled in their youth and dead by age 30. The recent development of a synthetic molecule that can correct the gene mutation causing the disease holds promise for victims.

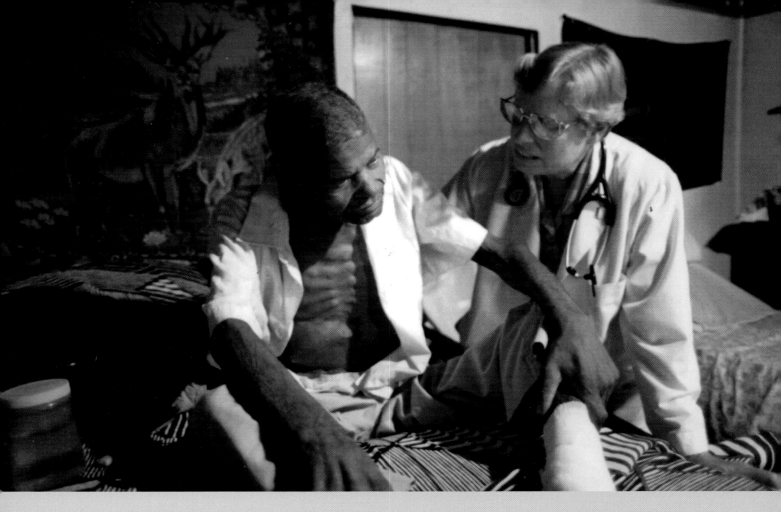

A Cancer Victim

*Jesse Morrisette, terminally ill
with esophageal cancer, is
comforted by Sister Roseanne,
who made a house call to see him.
Morrisette, 75, died a few weeks
after the photograph was made.*

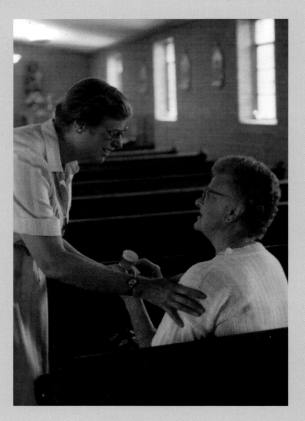

Mass Medication

*Sister Roseanne hands a prescription to patient
Mary Willingham before a Sunday morning
Mass at St. Joseph's Catholic Church in
Camden, Ala. Most of the church's 35
parishioners are members of Roman Catholic
orders who serve the poor in the region.*

when she "accepted the invitation of the Lord" and entered a convent 38 years ago in St. Louis. She earned her doctorate in developmental physiology and taught college-level biology. At age 40, again answering a call to serve the needs of society, she entered the University of Missouri–Columbia School of Medicine. After completing a family practice residency in 1986, she was recruited by fellow Sister Jane Kelly, a nurse practitioner, to join the clinic in Pine Apple, Ala. Sister Jane promised her "third world conditions," and that's what she found.

At the time, nearly half of the patients had no running water. More than 90 percent of them lived below the federal poverty level. More than half had no health insurance or government benefits.

Little has changed over the last decade. A rural water district now supplies part of the population. But many people, like Jesse Morrisette and Willie Reeds, can't afford to install plumbing.

"These are proud people who nearly always try to pay their bills one way or another," says Sister Roseanne. She's received fish, venison, corn, sweet potatoes and "most everything else."

Always upbeat, her friendly face framed by close-cropped strawberry blond hair and gold-rimmed glasses, Sister Roseanne is a tall, strong woman. Her sparkling blue eyes smile easily, and her toothy grin often leads to an infectious laugh as she talks lovingly about her patients.

"These are wonderful, warm people I serve," she says. "They give me countless intangible rewards. They work and help each other. We have no homeless here. They always have extra beds and food.

"They're at peace with their lot, which is poor. But they have lasting relationships, deep faith and a peacefulness you just can't buy. That's the real secret of Christmas."

Sister Roseanne sees about 30 patients daily at the Grace Busse Clinic in Pine Apple. The facility is partially funded by the U.S. Public Health Service. She lives 25 miles away in Camden with retired Sister Shirley Casler and several dogs and cats on Whiskey Run Road. She also cares for patients at the aging John Paul Jones Hospital in Camden, the county seat, where she shares on-call duties with the other three physicians who serve the county's 14,000 residents. She's racked up more than 300,000 miles over the past decade, "wearing out two cars and working on another one." Her compact Chevrolets are provided by her religious community, to which she signs over her $90,000 federal salary. She lives off a modest household budget provided by her order.

Sister Roseanne says she always feels safe in her solitary travels to see patients scattered throughout the pine woods of Wilcox County, where logging and hunting camps are primary industries. Even when she has car trouble, "Someone always comes along to help within a few minutes," she says.

The clinic is named for a Florida woman whose husband sent small

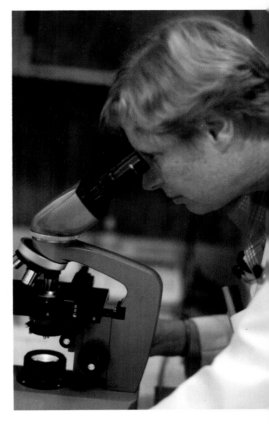

A Familiar Tool
Sister Roseanne uses a microscope in the small laboratory at her clinic. Before she became a family physician, she earned a doctorate in developmental physiology at Washington University in St. Louis and taught college biology.

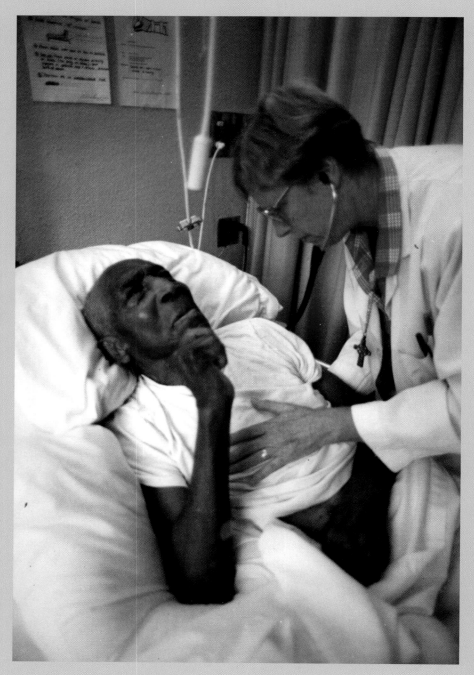

A Comforting Hand

Sister Roseanne comforts Melvin Stallworth, 86, a nursing home patient whose kidneys are failing, a few weeks before his death. She cared for him for nearly 10 years by making house calls to his tiny cabin, where he was wheelchair-bound.

donations to the nun after reading about her work in *McCall's* magazine. When his wife died of cancer in 1991, John Busse gave $50,000 in her memory, enough to renovate the dilapidated building that formerly served as a black school. Busse died within the year without ever having seen the clinic. Photos of the couple hang in the entrance hall. Their children and grandchildren continue to send money.

Besides the small clinic, the building now houses a learning center for tutoring of slow students and enrichment of the gifted, a nutrition unit that serves 25 meals a day, and day care for elderly and mentally retarded adults. There's also a new building for a thrift store and lunch room. These services are overseen by other nuns working with the missions of the Fathers of St. Edmund, a Vermont-based Catholic order that began work in Alabama in 1937.

Many patients can't afford to buy medicine. So Sister Roseanne hands out free medication she gets from charity sources and drug companies. Affluent physicians and hospitals send her medical supplies. She's always alert for new sources.

Her waiting room serves as a social gathering place for the community. People drop by just to see who's there and visit a bit, their chatter interrupted by the office nurse calling out patient names Southern style: "Miss Angenetta, Miss Gentsie, Mr. Melvin," and so on.

Common illnesses—hypertension, diabetes and cardiovascular conditions—stem from poor diet and obesity. And many mothers are reluctant to breast-feed because of the stigma attached to the earlier practice of blacks serving as "nurse maids" for white children.

When Hurricane Opal swept into South Alabama in October of 1995, Sister Roseanne closed her clinic early that day and made house calls to see two cancer patients. When both died later in the night during the height of the storm, relatives called her immediately. She made her way back to each home and sat with the families by lantern light until the undertaker arrived.

"It was eerie," she remembers. "It seemed as if the wind was carrying the patients' spirits with it. It moved me very much that, during such a terrible upheaval of the earth, this would be the time the Lord would take these people back. As the wind subsided, they just sort of drifted away to Him."

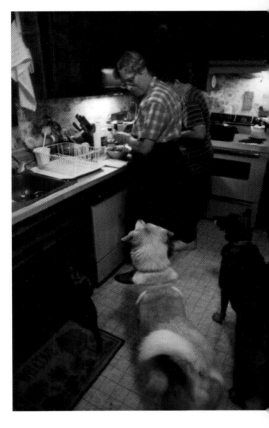

Chow Time
With their house pets waiting for a handout, Sister Roseanne and Sister Shirley Casler prepare supper at the convent in Camden, the Wilcox County seat where they live.

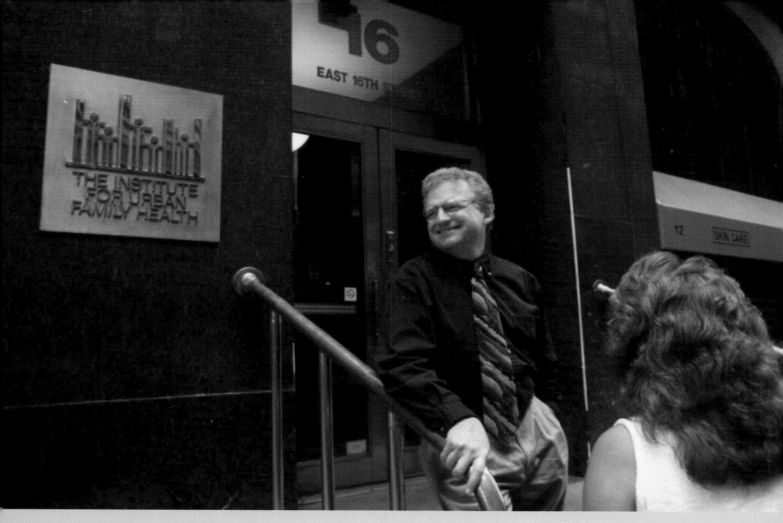

Street Talk

Calman talks to an employee as he stands on the steps of the Institute for Urban Family Health in Manhattan.

A Weight Problem

Calman examines Juan Martinez, 67, who came to the Bronx-Lebanon Hospital Outpatient Clinic complaining of chest and back pains. Calman suggested that losing weight might make him feel better. Martinez, a native of Honduras, moved to the United States in 1944. He retired after nearly 40 years working as an oiler aboard ships in the U.S. Merchant Marine Service.

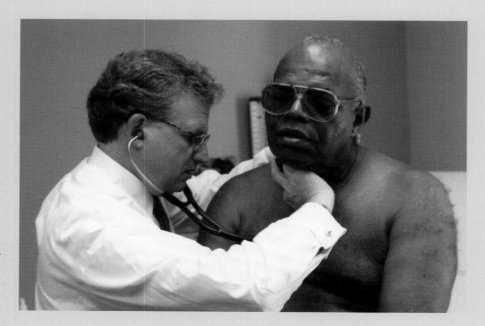

A Social Activist With a Stethoscope

Neil R. Calman, M.D.
New York City

eil Calman, M.D., 47, is a physician with a mission. Simply stated, his mission is to provide affordable health care to the thousands of underserved residents of New York City's boroughs. That's a tough assignment in some tough neighborhoods.

As a founder and president of the Institute for Urban Family Health, Calman oversees 350 employees and an $18 million (1996) annual budget. The not-for-profit institute bases its health services on the care provided by family physicians. Most of its projects operate in cooperation with community-based organizations, hospitals and medical schools.

The diminutive Calman's infectious enthusiasm seems to magnify his physical presence as he excitedly describes his work in the city he loves. When a first-time visitor to the South Bronx sees only razor wire–enclosed parking lots and graffiti-splashed buildings, Calman keeps up a steady commentary on neighborhood improvements. While his guest keeps an eye on the drug dealers and other people of the street, he offers unfettered optimism about future development.

Calman grew up in New York in a Jewish family, the son and grandson of dentists who also were social activists. "My grandfather was my biggest inspiration," Calman recalls. "He was a dentist, an attorney and a Socialist city alderman. He was a human rights person, one of those people who just lived his values.

"My dad followed in his footsteps, opening up a dental practice in a neighborhood that was all Jewish when he moved in and all minority, mostly black and Hispanic, when he moved out 40 years later. He adjusted to changes and just kept practicing there."

Calman's grandfather, a staunch supporter of organized labor, died while union gravediggers were on strike. Rather than cross picket lines and bury him in a grave dug by scab labor, the family had his body embalmed and refrigerated. They buried him after the walkout ended, Calman says with a laugh.

As a teen-ager, Calman spent summers as a medical research intern alongside a hematologist friend of his father. "That was a special thing. I thought I wanted to become a medical researcher," he recalls.

After earning an undergraduate degree from the University of Chicago in 1971, Calman went to the Rutgers Medical School with research his major interest. "I had just come out of the '60s with this social streak I'd grown up with. When I wasn't plugging away in the research lab, I was out protesting about something: better housing, jobs. When someone said I should just

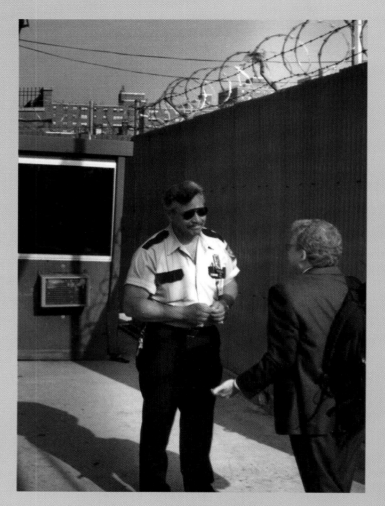

A Lot of Security
Calman visits with a guard at the razor wire–enclosed physicians parking lot at Bronx-Lebanon Hospital–Fulton Division in the South Bronx.

HIV Patient
A dejected Blaine Steele, 36, who has been diagnosed as HIV-positive, is reassured by Calman at the Sidney Hillman Family Practice Center in Manhattan. Steele, a security supervisor in the Bowery neighborhood, feared he was coming down with pneumonia again. "It feels like the flu. I think it's coming slowly," he said.

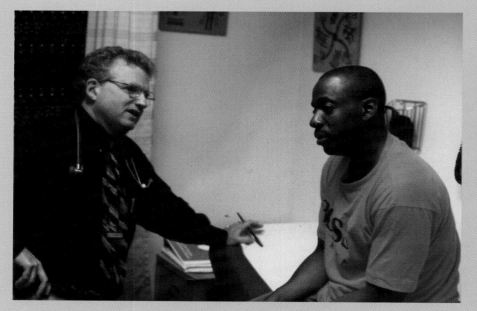

become a 'real' doctor instead of a researcher, I realized that two divergent parts of my life were coming together: The ability to do the science and medicine along with my social interests and commitment."

Calman began working as a volunteer in a primary-care clinic, and the experience changed his life. "I discovered I liked taking care of people who desperately needed it," says Calman, who never entered a medical research lab again.

Later, during his clinical years of medical school at Rush University in Chicago, he took a leave of absence for two months and worked with a family physician in a United Farm Workers health clinic in the grape fields of Southern California. "It was an incredible experience," he says. "We served people who had no other source of health care." Calman knew then he wanted to become a family doctor—in an urban area.

After graduation, he returned to New York and entered the family practice residency at Montefiore Medical Center. He picked Montefiore because the training was in Morrisania Hospital and Bathgate Health Center, both in the heart of the deteriorating South Bronx. During his residency, city officials closed Morrisania Hospital and bulldozed the Bathgate center and eight square blocks around it because the neighborhood seemed beyond repair. Calman and his fellow residents protested the closings. They had to complete their programs at another facility in the North Bronx in a much more upscale atmosphere.

Now, some 20 years later, Calman feels vindicated. His organization is playing a major role in the rebirth of the neighborhood. The institute's Crotona Park and Parkchester family practice clinics serve residents of low-income housing complexes in the rehabilitated Bathgate neighborhood. Both are modern, tastefully decorated facilities offering the latest in outpatient care.

The majestic Morrisania Hospital, a Bronx landmark since the 1920s, opens again this year as Urban Horizons, a $23 million renewal project that will provide housing, day care, job training—and one of Calman's family practice clinics to take care of the residents.

By building what he calls "gorgeous clinics in very poor neighborhoods," Calman accomplishes two major goals: "We give our patients the best possible care, which they deserve, in the best possible setting. It's so much better than the treatment they've had in the past in the emergency rooms of large institutions. And the nice clinics help us tremendously in recruiting and retaining the best family physicians. We are competitive in salaries, but we must give them decent environments in which to work."

Calman's approach offers physicians an opportunity to fulfill their social desires to care for the poor while still making a respectable professional living in decent surroundings. Calman says there's never been a violent incident or security problem at any of the clinics: "It's taboo. People are proud of what they have."

The institute is based at 16 E. 16th St., just off Union Square in downtown Manhattan, home of the Sidney Hillman Family Practice Center. The center, a

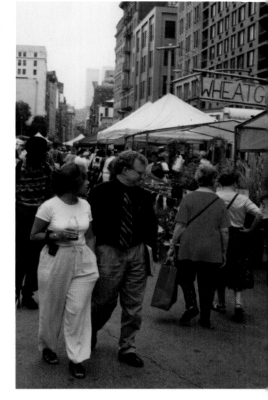

A Noon Stroll
Calman and companion Mayra Destefano walk through an outdoor market in Manhattan's Union Square during their lunch break. When Calman helped open the Institute for Urban Family Health a few doors away 10 years ago, an unethical doctor was handing out prescription drugs to addicts across the street. Storefronts were boarded up. Now, the "drug doctor" is gone, businesses are flourishing and two of New York's best restaurants are located there, Calman says.

comprehensive family practice clinic, houses the Beth Israel Medical Center Department of Family Medicine and Residency in Urban Family Practice, the first such facilities in a Manhattan hospital. The institute also operates a family practice residency program at Bronx-Lebanon Hospital in its efforts to increase the number of family physicians interested in inner city practice.

Calman, who still sees patients some days despite the crush of administrative duties, is the 1997 president of the New York State Academy of Family Physicians. He sees managed care as the "ideal solution" to providing health services to the underserved in the future. He also supports a national health plan to serve the entire nation. The institute recently started its own prepaid ABC Health Plan designed to better serve Medicaid recipients.

In addition to its eight family practice clinics, the institute operates eight small clinics at homeless shelters. Calman and most of his employees speak fluent Spanish because they serve so many Hispanic patients. Plans are on the drawing board to develop health services for new immigrants.

Neil Calman has been recognized with three major national awards for his innovative efforts in the past. When symptoms of new health-care ills show up among New York City's underserved in coming years, Calman is positioned well to make the diagnosis. His treatment plan no doubt will include a dose of good medicine mixed with social concern.

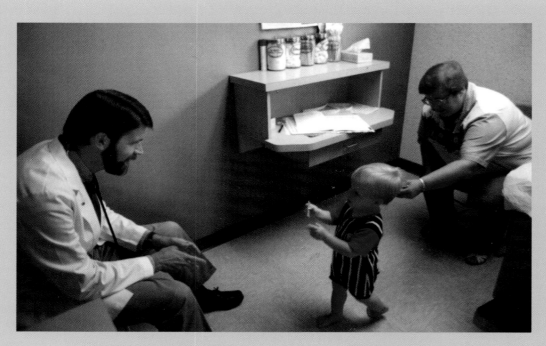

Gum for the Doctor
Seth Richardson, 2, takes a piece of gum to McRay at the prompting of his grandmother, Ritter Faulkner. She brought the toddler to the clinic with a rash from an apparent allergic reaction. His parents are Mitchael and Ethel Richardson.

A Ministry of Medicine in Appalachia

David McRay, M.D.
Jellico, Tennesee

*I*nspired to pursue a career in medicine by the family physician who delivered him, David McRay, M.D., 37, is now living his dream of "a ministry through medicine" in the mountains of Appalachia.

McRay and his family make their home in Jellico, Tenn., a depressed former coal-mining community that straddles the Tennessee-Kentucky border north of Knoxville. As medical director of three government-supported clinics, he oversees the primary care of more than 15,000 patients in one of America's poorest regions.

Born in 1960 in Searcy, Ark., McRay developed an early affection for Thomas Formby, M.D., whom he describes as a "mildmannered, loving, Christian man." Though McRay was only 5 when his family left Searcy, Formby's gentle influence was lasting. McRay has taken his family to Arkansas to meet Formby, who is retired.

McRay's father, an ordained Churches of Christ minister, eventually moved his family to Murfreesboro, Tenn., where David met another 14-year-old, a girl named Joan. Eight days after each graduated from college in Nashville—David at Vanderbilt and Joan at nearby George Peabody—they were married and left immediately for Chicago. David was bound for medical school at Northwestern University. Joan taught in the inner city to help pay their bills. She now home-schools their three young children, Jonathan, Michael and Anna, in their cozy old house on a hillside in Jellico.

While there are some tidy homes and well-kept churches, things are not well in Jellico, a village of 2,500 nestled between Pine and Indian mountains. Most of the mining jobs are gone. Unemployment pushes 25 percent. About 75 percent of the people in Campbell County get government assistance. Three-fourths of the residents smoke, three times the national average.

Indian Mountain Clinic in Jellico, where McRay practices, is one of three operated by Laurel Fork–Clear Fork Health Centers, Inc., the first federally funded community health entity in Tennessee. The other two clinics are in Clairfield, Tenn., and Williamsburg, Ky. The organization is the outgrowth of financially troubled clinics dating to the early 1950s.

McRay came to Jellico in 1989, intending to pay off his $60,000 medical school debt by working the required three years in the National Health Service Corps. The program is designed to attract young physicians to underserved regions. He saw such a fertile opportunity to serve that he stayed.

Colleagues credit McRay's personal sacrifice and leadership with keeping the clinics going when the Tenncare (Medicaid) organization failed to meet its

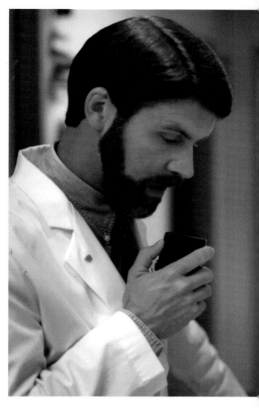

Chart Dictation
McRay dictates a patient chart at his Indian Mountain Clinic in Jellico, Tenn., on the Kentucky border. He was named the 1995 Tennessee Family Physician of the Year by the Tennessee Academy of Family Physicians.

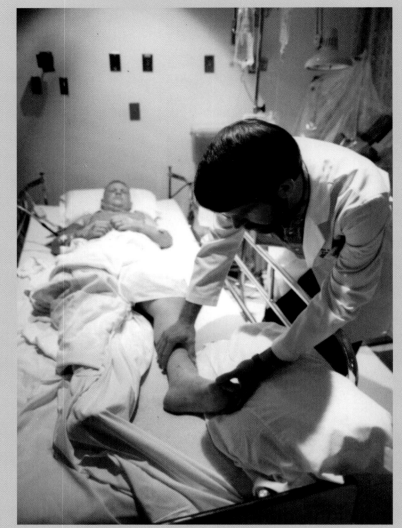

Snakebite Victim

Joey Jones, 14, is checked by McRay after a poisonous copperhead snake bit his foot near the family home on Westborne Mountain the night before. Jones was admitted to Jellico Community Hospital's intensive care unit as a precaution after antivenin was administered. "He was bad scared because I was panicky," his mother said. "We tied a string around his leg and drove to town in 14 minutes. It normally takes 35 minutes."

It's a Girl

McRay conducts an obstetrical ultrasound procedure on Bonnie Huff, one of his office employees. Two weeks later, she gave birth to Bryana Elizabeth, who weighed 6 pounds and 15 ounces. The family physician teaches OB ultrasound technique at medical schools in the region.

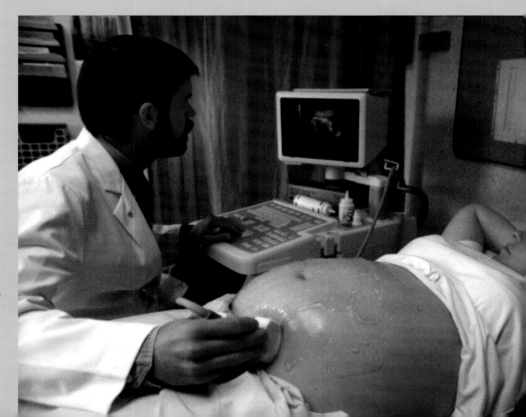

financial obligations in the early 90's. Serving for a year as executive director, McRay took a $27,000 personal salary cut. His example prompted the other staffers to contribute another $72,000 in salary reductions to ensure the survival of the operation. In 1996, McRay and other professionals worked for about 40 percent less than normal.

The U.S. Public Health Service annually provides a third of the clinics' $2.2 million budget. As many as 40 percent of the patients live below poverty level. Nearly 85 percent of them receive some form of government-paid health care or have no insurance at all.

McRay performs a wide range of patient services, including Caesarean sections, and is known for his expertise in obstetric ultrasound procedures.

The 54-bed Jellico Community Hospital, operated by the Seventh Day Adventist Church, provides inpatient services for the region.

Deeply committed to his Christian faith, McRay first considered a career as a medical missionary in Central America, where he has served on medical teams five times. But he and Joan decided to return and serve the mountain people they knew.

"We've tried to recruit doctors to Jellico who come because they want to be a part of this ministry. We've got a core group like that, but we've not been able to attract enough to make the health center stable," McRay says. "So we have to rely on doctors willing to stay just two or three years."

The physician says his faith is at the core of why he has stayed in Jellico. "For many years I dreamed of and felt called to a life of ministry through medicine," he says. "My personal commitment to living and working among the poor is the result of my faith. That's why I'm in family practice. It's a common day for me to go from bringing a child into the world to dealing with an elderly patient approaching death.

"Being involved in all those major life events is what makes family practice unique. It's being able to touch the lives of my patients at those critical moments.

"So many of the problems people face are really spiritual illnesses that manifest themselves as physical ailments. Depression, anxiety and a lot of other things can come from spiritual unrest. We talk with our patients and pray with them, and I think we help them a lot."

He is aware of a "fair amount" of promiscuity in an area where sexually transmitted diseases are common. But the region is so isolated that McRay saw only two cases of HIV in his first seven years. Hard-core substance abuse is not as prevalent either. Alcohol, tobacco and marijuana rank as the biggest drug problems.

"With the culture of poverty seen in Appalachia come things like broken families, high teen-age pregnancy, and alcohol and tobacco abuse, leading to significant health problems, such as artery disease and chronic lung disease, among people who have worked in the mines," McRay observes.

He attributes his successes to the close partnership he and his wife have

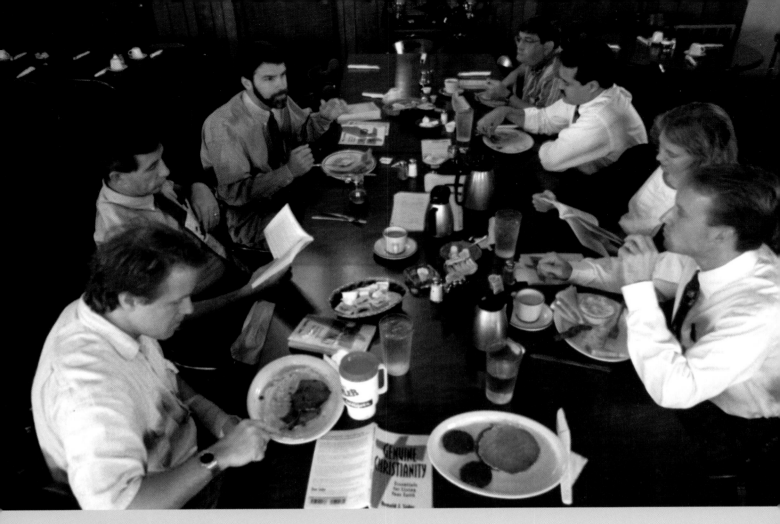

The Christian Focus

McRay (in blue shirt) and other Indian Mountain Clinic staffers, all devout Christians, meet at a Jellico restaurant for their weekly Friday morning prayer breakfast. The discussion, based on a book titled Genuine Christianity *by Ronald J. Sider, centered on family values and the responsibility of community members to preserve and strengthen marriages and family environments.*

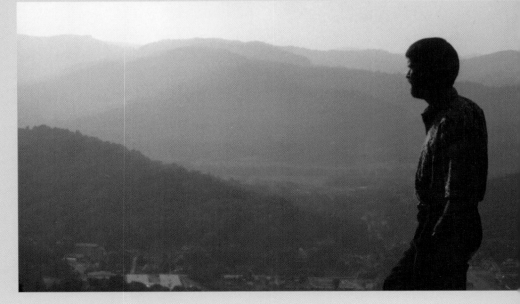

Inspirational View

McRay is silhouetted against the Cumberland Mountains, where many of his patients live, as he enjoys a sunset at a favorite spot on Pine Mountain. The community of Jellico is visible below him.

developed. "We are a traditional family by choice. Early on, we both agreed that she would stay home and raise our kids. The things I've accomplished in medicine and church and community have been possible only because we've worked as a team. From home-schooling to managing the household, she's made it all possible," McRay says appreciatively.

"Having a family, to me, is critical to being a good family physician," he continues. "Understanding family dynamics and what goes on in the process of raising kids is crucial. As the kids get older, I have come to understand the real necessity of my presence at home. I'm scaling back my professional activities and trying to find out what it really means to put God first, family second and work third, advice Dr. Formby has given me for years.

"He always said to be careful about medicine: It has its way of working to the top of that list. It's a growth process for me to realize that the next 10 years with my kids are vital. As important as my medicine and ministry are, when I get to the end of those 10 years, I want to look back and say I was there and I did the right thing for my family."

Those who know David McRay have no doubts that he will do the right thing.

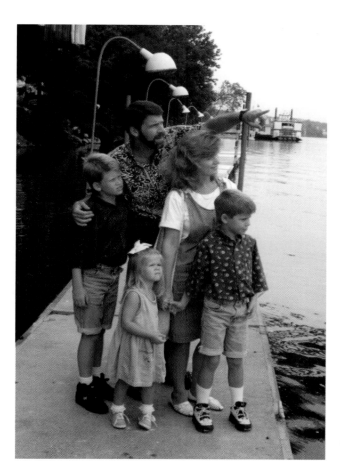

A Family Outing
The McRay family enjoys the Tennessee River at a restaurant in Knoxville, where the physician spent a Saturday morning in a continuing medical education class. With McRay are his wife, Joan, and children Jonathan, left, Anna and Michael.

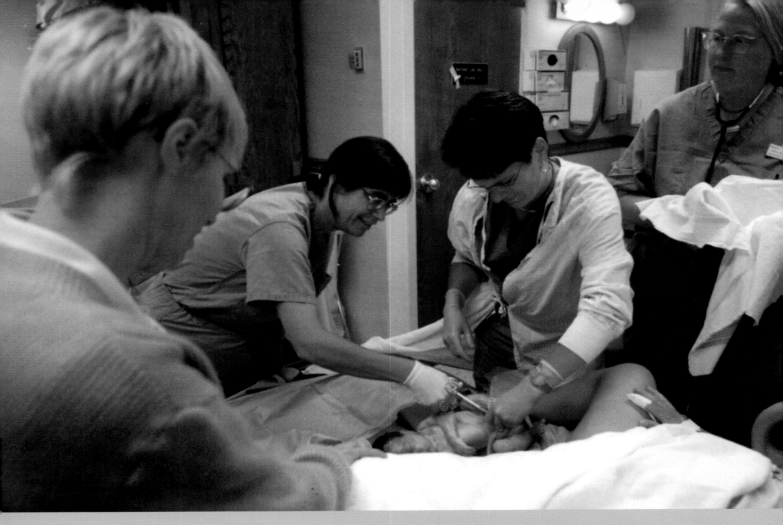

Welcome to the World

Corral snips the umbilical cord on Emil Benjamin Alspaugh after he was delivered by Suzanne Welsch, M.D. (in white coat), an obstetrics resident at the University of Utah Medical Center. At left is family friend Linda Ballard. The parents, Elena and Kevin Alspaugh, are Corral's patients. Formerly homeless, they now have their own apartment, and Kevin is enrolled in college.

Homeless and Paralyzed

Corral comforts a homeless drug addict in a Salt Lake City hospital. The 42-year-old man became paralyzed from the chest down after a fall. He could speak only in a whisper.

A Medical Mom:
Surviving Stress in Salt Lake

Silvia Corral, M.D.
Salt Lake City

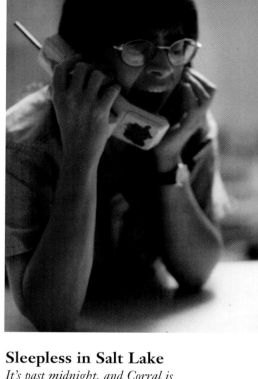

*S*ilvia Corral, M.D., 43, seldom hears her alarm clock. She usually is awakened about 6:30 a.m. by 3-year-old twins Tomas and Isabel or brother Benjamin, 6.

Corral is a single mother who is juggling the crush of child-raising with her demanding career as a family physician running a clinic for the homeless in Salt Lake City. Coping with family schedules and finances was easier when she was married, but she works hard to make the best of her situation.

Breakfast for Mom and kids is cold cereal and juice. Then it's time to wash faces, brush teeth, dress and gather security blankets, toys and lunch pails. All four are still tired from a wonderful family roughhouse on the floor the night before.

By 8:30, Mom leads a Pied Piper troupe out the door singing, "Hi ho, hi ho, it's off to work we go." She aims her blue Subaru wagon out of the subdivision, down the long hill past the majestic Utah Capitol Building and toward Benjamin's Montessori school two miles away. The twins, still sleepy and snug in their car seats, wait while Mom escorts Benjamin safely inside for a discreet goodbye hug.

Tomas and Isabel ride across town with Mom to join several other children in private day care. After hugs and words of encouragement about their day, the twins are content to stay.

As medical director of the 4th Street Clinic for the homeless, Silvia Corral never knows what the day will bring. But her life experiences have prepared her.

Sleepless in Salt Lake
It's past midnight, and Corral is on call covering patients in four hospitals. Yawning, she returns a phone call from her home before going to bed. Two hours later, she was summoned by pager to deliver a baby.

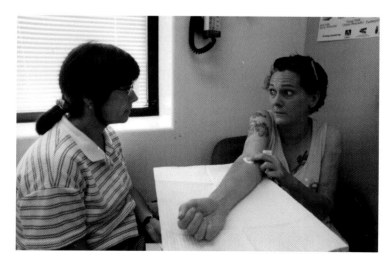

Fighting Addiction
Sherri Bodily, 38, a recovering addict who is receiving Methadone treatments, discusses her problems with Corral at the 4th Street Clinic for the homeless.

95

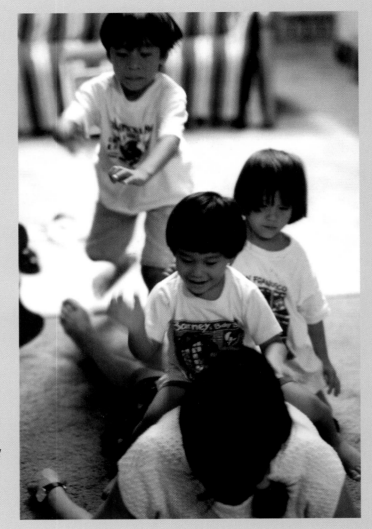

Romping With Mom

Benjamin, 6, is about to throw his full weight into a bedtime roughhouse with Mom and 3-year-old twins Tomas and Isabel on the family room floor. Corral's children are her first priority. She plans her practice around their needs.

A Homeless Iguana

Corral stops on the street in front of Salt Lake City's biggest indigent shelter to talk to a homeless boy about his pet iguana, which he parked on her shoulder. Other members of the boy's family are nearby.

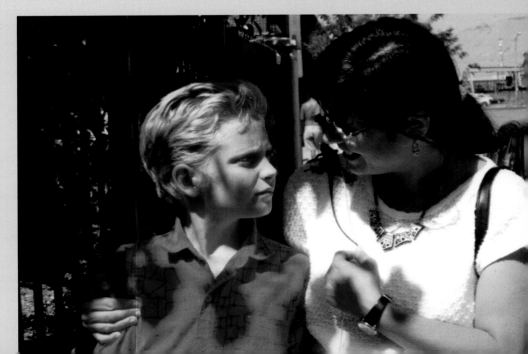

She and three siblings were born to poor Mexican-American farm workers who had settled in Santa Barbara, Calif. By 1966, her hard-working parents had saved enough money to return to Mexico, always their dream. Silvia, then 12, announced she was staying in the United States to live with an aunt and continue the schooling she dearly loved. Her parents relented and eventually became American citizens.

"I was a gifted student. I called it my gift from God. I knew my future in Mexico would be to get married and make tortillas," Corral says. After high school, Stanford University gave her a good financial aid package. She graduated in four years, "always praying to God before my tests," with two degrees and a 3.86 grade point average, and was accepted into the Stanford School of Medicine.

After a three-year family practice residency, she worked part time as an emergency room physician while she earned a master's degree in public health at the University of California, Los Angeles..

"My mother always loved her doctors. We took special food and flowers to them every Christmas. She instilled in me that they were people to be appreciated and respected. That's where I got my sense of what a physician means to people," Corral explains.

It's nearly 9 a.m., and Silvia Corral's day as a doctor begins. She shifts gears in the station wagon and stabs the keys on her cellular phone to find out where she needs to go first. One of her transient patients is not doing well at Salt Lake Regional Health Center. Arriving on the patient's floor, Corral talks to a concerned family practice resident. The patient, who fell at a nursing home several days earlier, has undergone neurosurgery. Now he's paralyzed from the neck down. Something obviously has gone wrong. The man, a longtime drug addict at age 42, can only whisper. He begs Corral for an extra prescription of Percodan, a powerful narcotic. She refuses.

Then she's off to the University of Utah Medical Center to check on a maternity patient. The woman is having problems, and Corral makes the decision to induce labor. The patient and her husband formerly were homeless. The man is now a college student, and they have their own apartment, a success story Corral is proud of.

She heads back across town, along familiar streets, with Corral using the cell phone again. She stops at the Utah Department of Health and consults with a supervisor in the Ethnic Health Work Force Program. Corral works fervently as an advocate for better health care for the underserved. Last year she chaired the Salt Lake City-County Health Department board.

At 11:20 a.m., she drives to her 4th Street Clinic, in the Rio Grande neighborhood where many of Salt Lake City's thousands of homeless people stay. Rio Grande is a haven for the homeless because of its network of shelters, soup kitchens and other social services that accommodate hundreds daily.

Transients are drawn from all over the West. Many sleep in the open in nearby Pioneer Park.

The 4th Street Clinic provides these people with a medical home. The comprehensive health-care facility is funded by federal monies for homeless health care and private donations. Other agencies assist, along with some 200 volunteer professional health-care providers.

"A lot of homeless people are sick. If not, they certainly deserve to be kept healthy," Corral says. "We give them all the types of care they could get anywhere else." The clinic does a lot of nutrition education and screenings for cholesterol, diabetes, AIDS, other sexually transmitted diseases and tuberculosis.

In early afternoon, Corral joins staffers she has invited from a local hospital to tour the huge Travelers Aid Society shelter. As they leave her clinic, bicycle-mounted police are rousting three young transients loitering in front. One cop mutters, "These people are animals." Corral is furious, but says nothing.

Back inside the clinic, she tends to administrative duties and sees patients for a couple of hours. One is a recovering addict on a methadone program. Another is a homeless woman who hurt her shoulder in a warehouse job.

It's late afternoon, and Corral has forgotten to eat lunch. She's on call through the night. Her former husband, a research physician, will pick up the children and keep them overnight and the next day. She drives to a nursing home to examine and sign release papers for a professional man whose chronic alcoholism has ruined his health. He's going to try again to see whether he can live in an apartment.

Miraculously, Corral manages to spend nearly two hours enjoying a leisurely dinner at the home of friends before her pager sounds. She's needed to deliver a baby at Salt Lake Regional. After an hour, the patient's doctor arrives and takes over. Corral is paged to another hospital. She discovers a patient has gone without needed IV medication for several hours. That upsets her.

At 12:30 a.m., Corral arrives home and listens to several phone messages before going to bed. The pager wakes her at 2:25. The patient whose labor was induced finally is about ready to deliver at the university medical center. Corral dresses quickly and races the Subaru through dark streets to the hospital. Emil Benjamin Alspaugh, 7 pounds 14 ounces, finally arrives at 4:42 a.m.

At 6:30 a.m., the weary doctor is back home for a shower and change of clothes as she prepares for another day.

On paper, Corral works only 60 percent regular hours to limit her on-call requirement. "Being a mommy has to come first," she says. "Caring for the underserved has special stresses from complex issues and a lack of resources. I bring all that home with me to add to my own family and financial stress."

It's not an easy life, but Silvia Corral probably wouldn't want to do anything else.

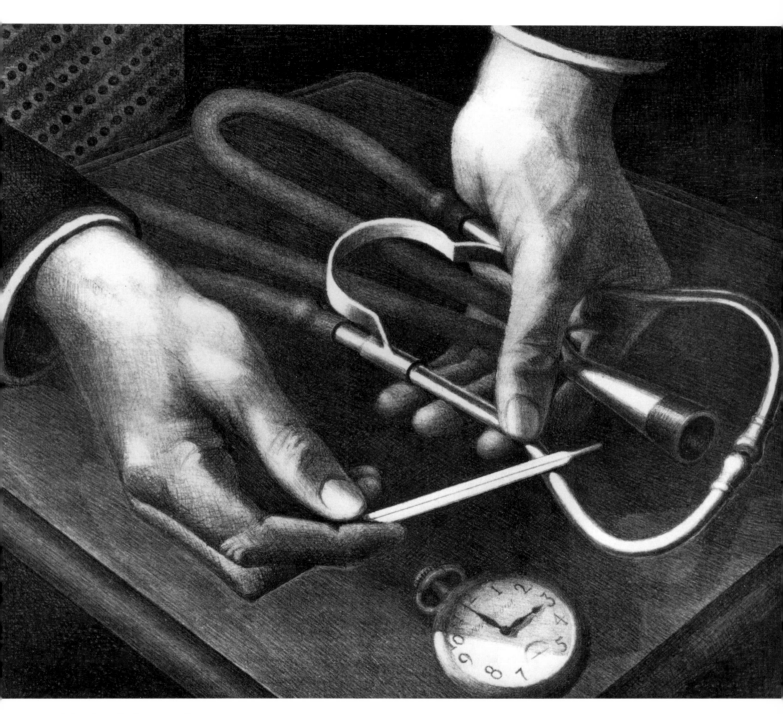

Tools of the Profession

Family Doctor, *a lithograph by Grant Wood, was produced in 1941, a year before
the famed Iowa artist died. A leader of the Regionalism school of art, his most famous
painting was* American Gothic. *(Cedar Rapids Museum of Art, gift of Harriet Y.
and John B. Turner II.)*

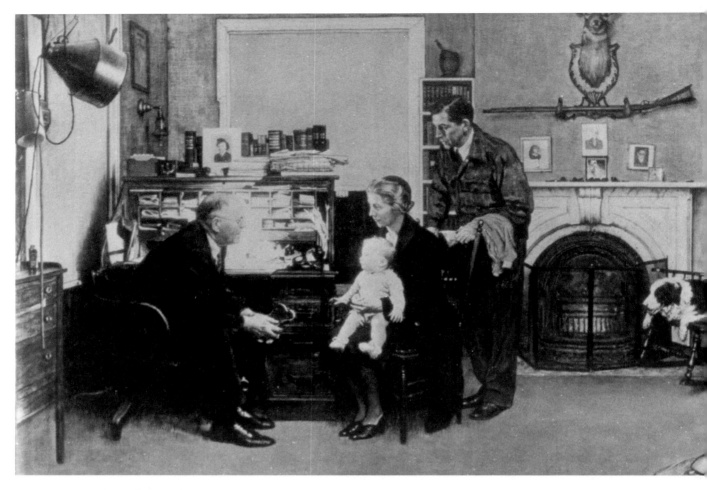

Norman Rockwell Visits a Family Doctor

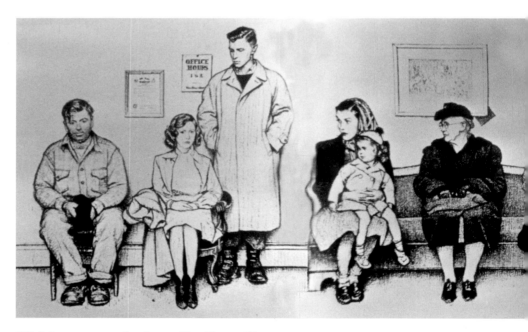

Waiting to see the busy Dr. Russell.

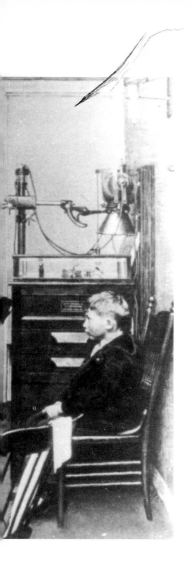

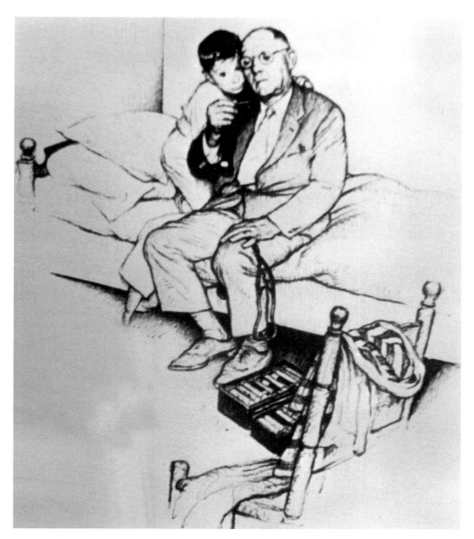

Bad news: "You may have to go back to school."

Rockwell Son Recalls Physician

Norman Rockwell Visits a Family Doctor and nine related sketches were published in the April 12, 1947, *Saturday Evening Post*. The physician is George A. Russell, M.D., who settled in 1911 in Arlington, Vt., where the Rockwell family lived in the late 1930s and '40s. His waiting room and office were in his fine old colonial home. Rockwell's son, Thomas Rockwell, remembers Dr. Russell "sitting on the edge of my bed with me" during house calls. Rockwell, 64, of Poughkeepsie, N.Y., laughs about another memory. "When I was a teen-ager I got a terrible shock while Dr. Russell was using his electric machine to burn off a wart. I must have been grounded." The younger Rockwell also recalls spending one high school summer in Dr. Russell's back rooms indexing his "marvelous collection of historical documents, pamphlets and books about Vermont." (Photos courtesy of The Norman Rockwell Museum at Stockbridge. Printed by permission of the Norman Rockwell Family Trust. Copyright 1943 the Norman Rockwell Family Trust.)

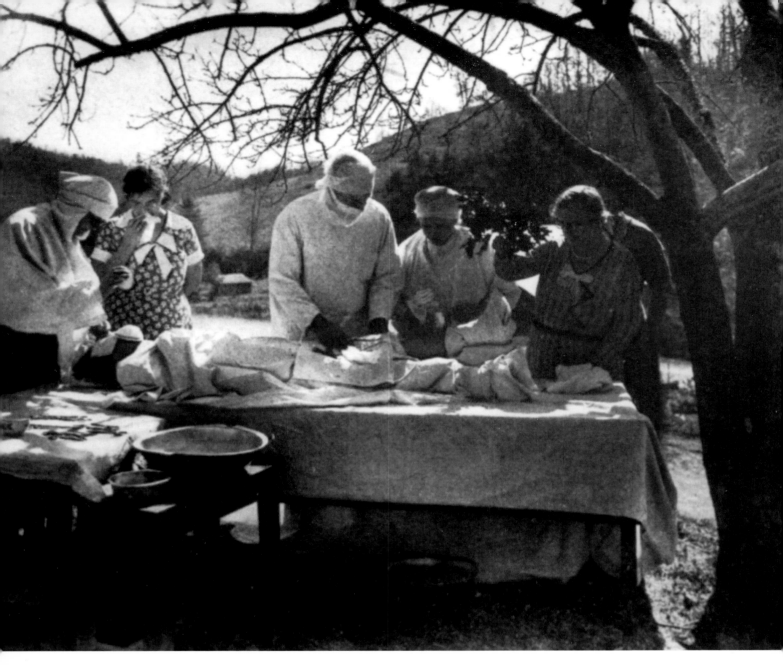

Antiseptic Apple Tree

Mary Martin Sloop, M.D., and her husband, Eustace Sloop, M.D., operate on a patient's leg under an apple tree, which they considered to be "the most antiseptic spot" in Crossnore, N.C., circa 1920. Later they helped found a hospital there. An assistant administers ether, and the woman at right fans flies away with a leafy branch. Mary Sloop, a 1906 graduate of the Woman's Medical College of Pennsylvania at Philadelphia, was named America's Mother of the Year at age 78 in 1951. She was a tireless crusader for better education for what she called "these fine mountain people." (North Carolina Division of Archives and History.)

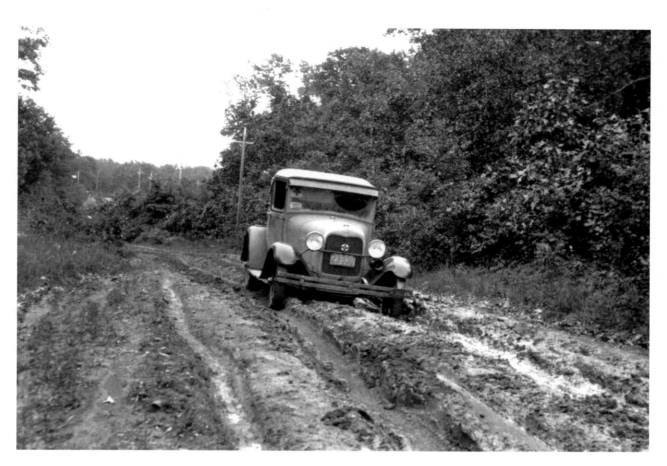

Following the Ruts

Muddy roads in June of 1931 didn't deter C.R. Macdonnell, M.D., from making his appointed rounds in his Model A Ford in rural Webster County, Missouri. Macdonnell, who lived in the Ozarks community of Marshfield, practiced in the region for nearly 40 years. See profile on his son, Tommy Macdonnell, M.D., in Chapter 3. (Tommy Macdonnell, M.D.)

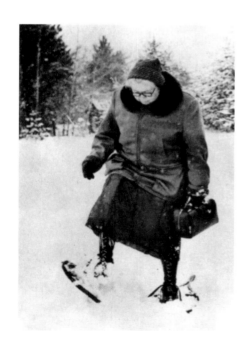

Winter in Wisconsin

Kate Newcomb, M.D., braves a snowstorm as she trudges along on snowshoes to make a house call somewhere in Wisconsin, circa 1927. (Andrew Pavelin, Chicago Tribune. *State Historical Society of Wisconsin. WHi{X3}24209.)*

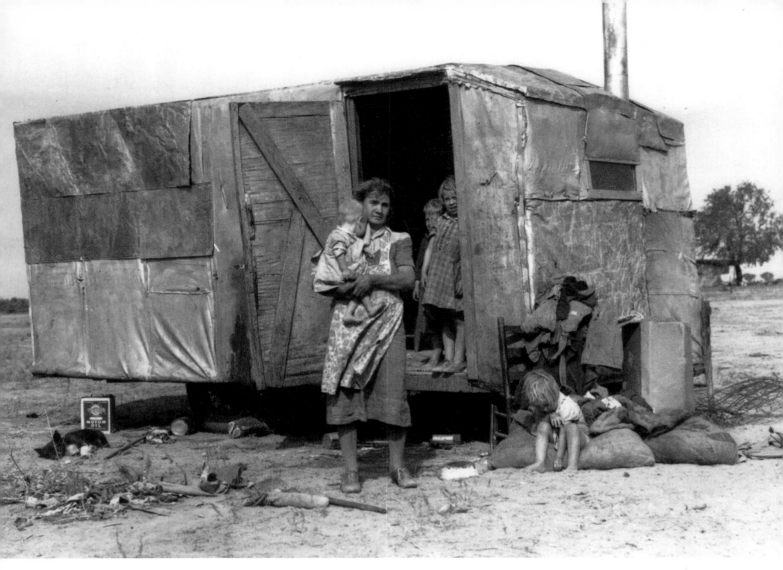

Migrant Family

Squalid living conditions, and resulting health problems, were common among migrant workers in 1940, when Dorothea Lange photographed this family along Arizona Highway 87 south of Chandler. Living with no water or sanitary facilities, they had come from Amarillo, picking cotton across Texas, New Mexico and Arizona. (National Archives. 83-G-44360.)

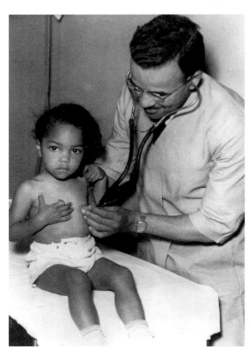

School Exam

J.W. Crump, M.D., conducts a health examination at a public school in St. Paul, Minn., circa 1940. Crump was active in assisting with Negro Health Week in the Twin Cities. (Minnesota Historical Society.)

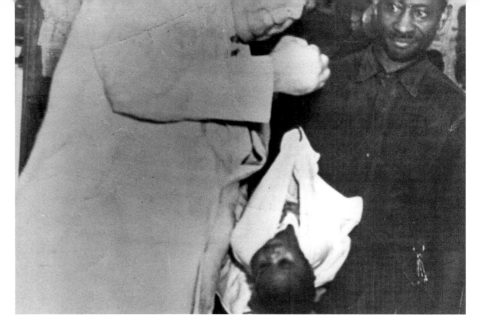

Record Book Baby

J.W. McPheeters, M.D., weighs a 20-pound baby girl in July of 1940 in his office at Poplar Bluff, Mo., as proud father Joe Hunter watches. Kathryn Hunter Slater, who was the largest newborn on record at the time, retired in 1994 after teaching school for 32 years near Harvey, Ill. She was her mother's 10th child. An older sibling weighed 14 pounds. (Roberts V. Stanard photo courtesy Lucy Lee Healthcare System.)

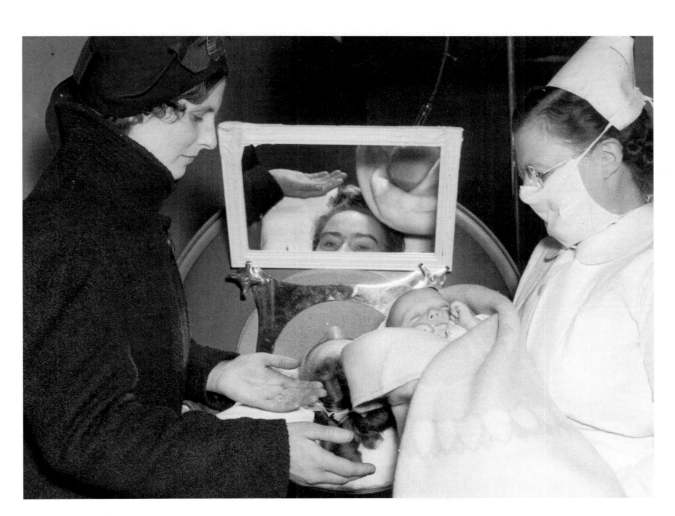

Iron Lung Patient

A nurse displays an infant to a polio patient in an iron lung breathing device, circa 1940, at the University of Minnesota Hospital in Minneapolis. The patient likely is the mother of the child. The woman at left, perhaps a family member, is unidentified. (Minnesota Historical Society.)

GIs Recuperating

Two wounded U.S. Army veterans of World War II's Battle of the Bulge in Europe recuperate at the Fort Crook, Neb., Army Hospital in the spring of 1945. The GI at left, identified only as "Quanna," is an American Indian from Oregon. A Nazi bullet blinded him in his right eye. (Nebraska State Historical Society.)

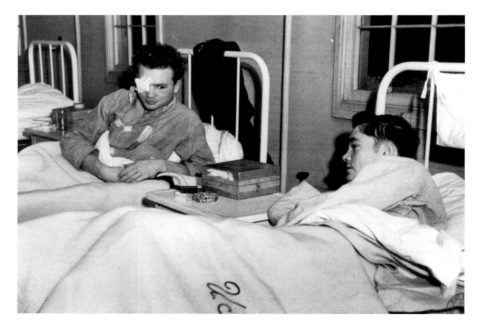

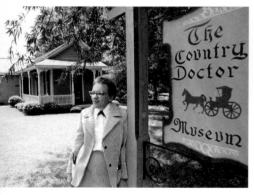

Museum Founder

Josephine E. Newell, M.D., at The Country Doctor Museum at Bailey, N.C., circa 1970. Newell, the seventh in a direct line of country doctors, founded the museum in 1968. The museum includes two old doctor offices that were moved to the site. It contains physicians' furniture and equipment, medical instruments, pharmaceutical displays and other memorabilia. (Bruce Roberts Collection. The Center for American History. The University of Texas at Austin. CN08897.)

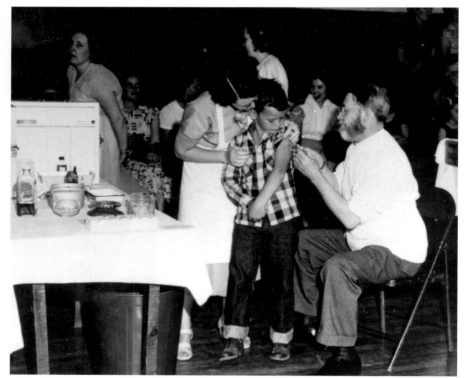

First Polio Shots

C.R. Macdonnell, M.D., gives a Salk polio vaccination to an apprehensive boy at Elkland, Mo., Elementary School on May 6, 1955. The 42 schoolchildren inoculated that day by Macdonnell and his son, Tommy Macdonnell, M.D., were the first in Missouri to receive the vaccine. (Tommy Macdonnell, M.D.)

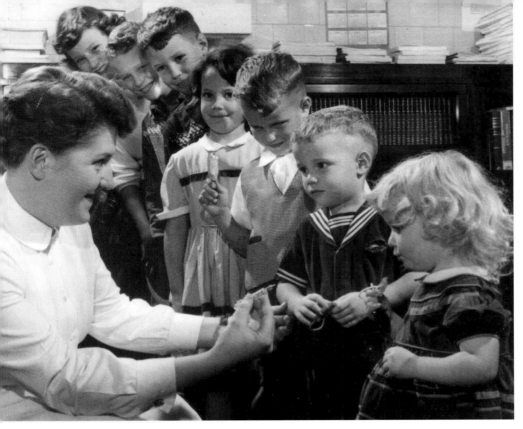

Calming Candy
Lollipops help pacify the seven children of Mrs. Paul Marnell of Milwaukee as they receive Salk polio inoculations from nurse Rosemarie Hernet on Nov. 15, 1955. (Milwaukee Journal. State Historical Society of Wisconsin. WHi(X3)43209.)

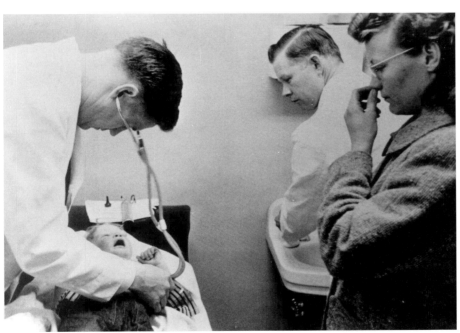

Learning Rural Medicine
H.P. "Pete" Ekern, left, a senior medical student at the University of Missouri in 1959, examines a protesting Darrell Carter as his mother, Mrs. D.E. Carter, watches. The diagnosis: Measles! Ekern spent six weeks living and working with family physician Tommy Macdonnell, M.D., (washing hands) in Webster County, Mo., to find out what rural practice was all about. Ekern returned to his hometown of Mexico, Mo., where he remains in active practice as a family physician. (Glenn Hensley, The Missouri Farmer. Courtesy University of Missouri–Columbia School of Medicine.)

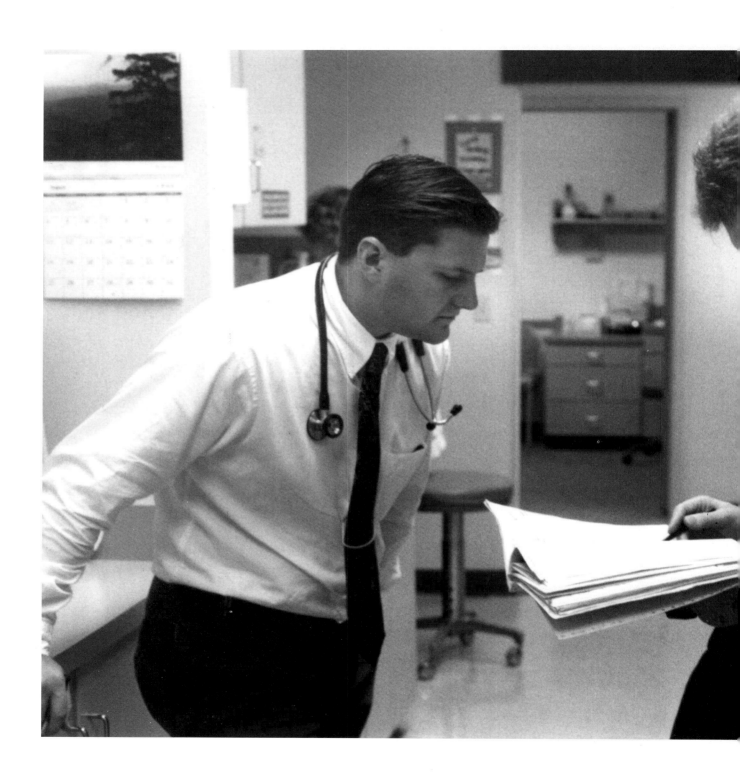

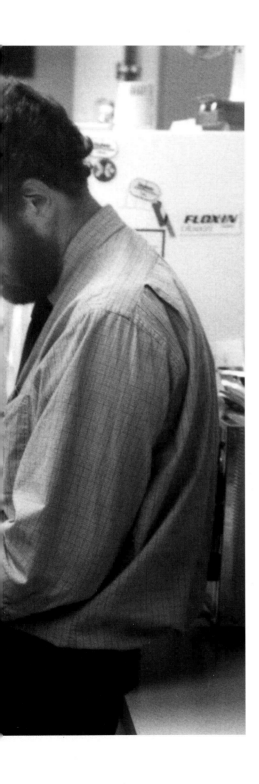

CHAPTER 4

Training Physicians for the Specialty

*Y*esterday's general practitioner and today's family physician share a commitment to caring for patients of all ages and both sexes, over time. The key difference is in the training: Yesterday's GP usually went into practice after a year of internship; any additional training was taught literally by the school of experience. Today's family physician, in contrast, benefits from three years of post–medical school training in a family practice residency.

Medical school graduates looking toward careers in family practice now have available more than 450 residencies for those three years of training. Some residencies are oriented to rural practice, while others focus on urban settings. Some do both.

A Quick Conference

Mark B. Schabbing, M.D., left, a second-year resident at the University of Missouri's family practice residency, waits to hear attending physician James Stevermer, M.D., comment on Schabbing's diagnosis of a patient's symptoms. Stevermer is an academic fellow and clinical instructor at the residency. The interaction takes place at the residency's Callaway Clinic in Fulton, Mo., the site of Schabbing's continuity practice, where he will care for many of the same patients for three years.

Family practice residencies are distinctive from residencies in any other specialty:

• Family practice residents are trained predominantly in an outpatient clinic setting called a "family practice center," giving them experience that closely mirrors actual practice.

• In the family practice center, residents see the same patients over time, in the context of the family and community, and must diagnose "undifferentiated" health problems—symptoms and complaints that may result from a number of different causes.

• Behavioral science training is mandatory for family practice residents, helping them learn how to establish effective relationships with their patients, as well as to understand the relationship of people's lives and symptoms.

One such program is the nationally recognized residency at the University of Missouri–Columbia School of Medicine, which has produced nearly 230 family physicians since it began in 1970 as one of the first in the country.

Though the Missouri program has a rural orientation, the largest of its three outpatient clinics is the Green Meadows Family Practice Center in Columbia. Green Meadows, which resembles a metropolitan multispecialty group practice, also is home to primary-care activities of the Departments of Obstetrics and Gynecology, Internal Medicine, and Child Health. The university's health maintenance organization (HMO) plan for employees is based at Green Meadows, giving residents practical experience working within a managed care setting.

Rural practice experience comes at either the Fayette Medical Clinic 30 miles northwest of Columbia or at Callaway Physicians, the residency's practice in Fulton, 25 miles to the east.

Fayette and Fulton are towns of 3,000 and 10,000, respectively, with economies based on agriculture and private colleges. Fulton has Callaway Community Hospital, where residents gain inpatient experience in addition to their work at the 400-bed University Hospital in Columbia. Fayette has no hospital, which challenges residents to learn to deal with hospitalizing patients (usually at University Hospital) from a remote clinic. Residents also can get more inpatient experience at a veterans hospital located in Columbia.

Residents select one of the three clinics as the site for a "continuity" practice and see the same patients at that site for three years. They also rotate to the other two sites to care for "walk-in" patients.

In addition, residents typically experience the following "rotations" during their training: emergency medicine, pediatrics, obstetrics and gynecology, internal medicine, geriatrics, newborn intensive care, well-baby nursery, orthopedics, ophthalmology, urology, ear-nose-throat, surgery, medical

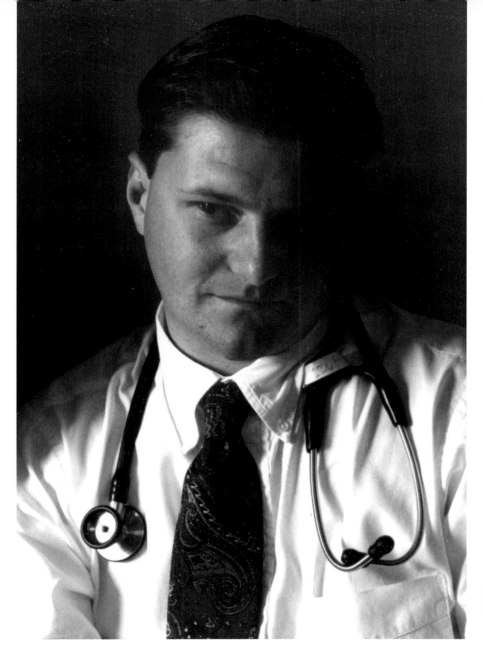

Thinking It Over

In a pensive moment, Schabbing reflects on his experiences at the end of a busy day at the clinic. The son of a Jackson, Mo., veterinarian, he plans to practice in a small town after completing his residency.

intensive care unit, cardiology, coronary care unit and dermatology. Some rotations are repeated, and there's time for several electives.

Each resident pairs off with a partner the first year of the program. The partners jointly assume patient care responsibilities in the clinic setting and on hospital rotations. Graduates say the partnership is one of the most important and gratifying parts of the MU residency. The experience of working with a partner provides an excellent model for future practice.

Residents also benefit from four day-long seminars on managing their future practices, planned and supervised by a faculty member with a master's degree in business administration who also has experience in private medical practice. They are paid a nominal salary and meal allowance, typically about one-third of the salary they'll receive when they enter practice.

Through the years, the Missouri program has had two goals, says Jack Colwill, M.D., professor and chairman of the Department of Family and

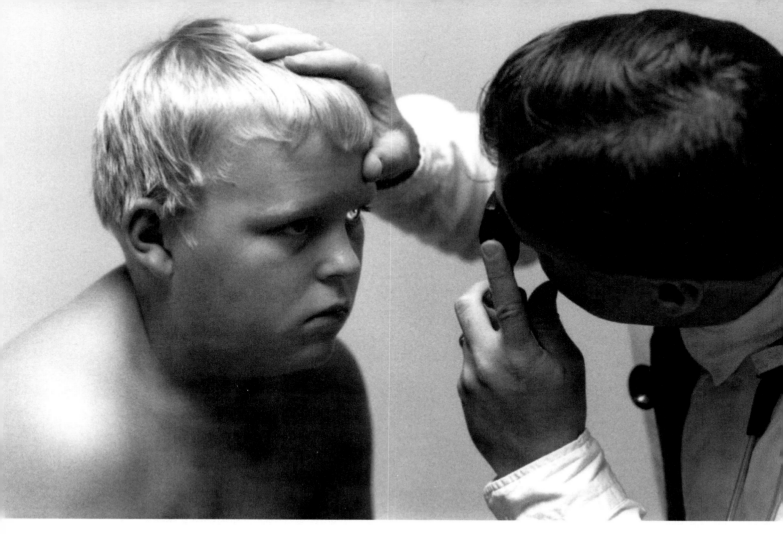

Sports Physical
Leslie Arms, 12, gets the required examination so he can play junior high school football. Leslie spent most of the summer hauling hay, and later played center at football camp. Schabbing promised the youth he always would be available to discuss in confidence any personal problems that might crop up. Leslie's reply, which pleased Schabbing: "I always talk to my parents if I have a problem."

Industrial Accident
Schabbing examines the hand of Terry Harrison, 48, who suffered a freeze burn when a seal broke on a propane tank at the refractory where he works in Fulton. The physician bandaged the hand, which did not appear to be seriously injured.

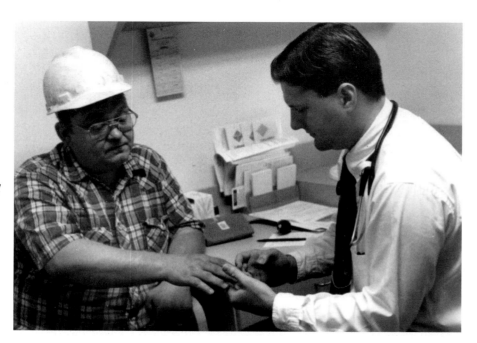

Community Medicine for the past quarter-century and a member of the prestigious Institute of Medicine of the National Academy of Sciences. "One is to prepare physicians who will be interested in small-town practice. The other is to train people for academic family medicine. There have been real shortages in both areas."

To date, the residency program has been highly successful in achieving both objectives. About 60 percent of its graduates have entered practice in small communities (twice the national average of all family practice residency graduates), and about 20 percent are full-time academics (five times the national average).

Nearly 90 percent have remained in some type of family practice career. A high percentage do obstetrics.

Missouri's Department of Family and Community Medicine also houses the $33 million Generalist Physician Initiative sponsored by the Robert Wood Johnson Foundation. Directed by Colwill and two MU associates, the initiative funds grants to 12 medical schools for programs to produce more generalist physicians—including family physicians, general internists and general pediatricians—who are increasingly in demand, especially with the growth of managed health care.

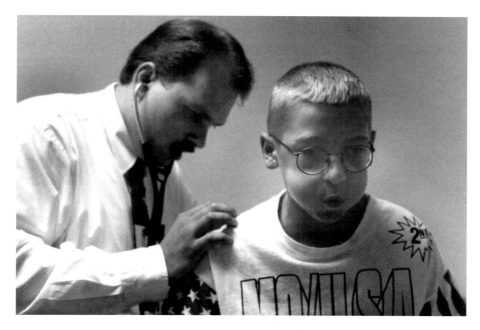

A Deep Breath

Matthew Lamons, 12, takes a deep breath for Jim R. Elam, M.D., who gives the youth a physical examination for seventh-grade sports. Matthew's goal is to play tight end on the football team. Elam, a native of Tulsa, Okla., is Schabbing's residency partner at the Fulton clinic.

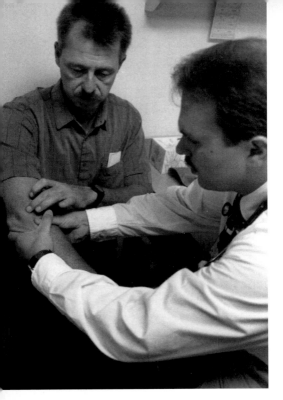

'Tennis Elbow'

Donald Racinowski, 40, comes to see Elam with painful tendonitis, which makes it difficult for him to work at his two jobs as a Fulton firefighter and commercial electrician. The condition commonly is called "tennis elbow."

Third-Year Resident

Shane Foster, M.D., relaxes for a few moments after seeing patients all morning at the Fayette, Mo., Medical Clinic, the site of his continuity practice. Foster, a native of Hickory, N.C., hopes to practice in his hometown after completing his residency.

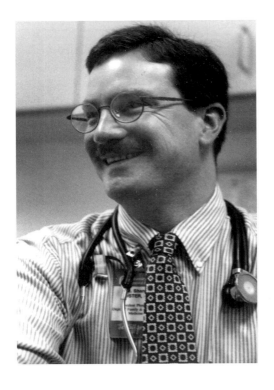

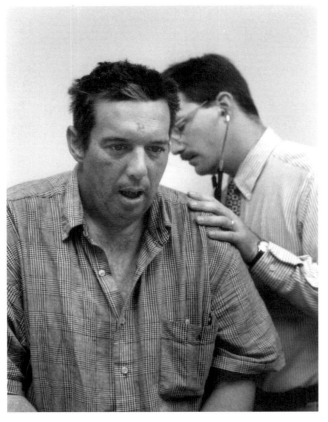

Lung Problems

Kevin Chandler, 34, a heavy smoker, comes to the Fayette Clinic with chronic bronchitis. Foster encouraged him to quit cigarettes. Chandler lives in a boarding home, where he receives help with medications for mental problems.

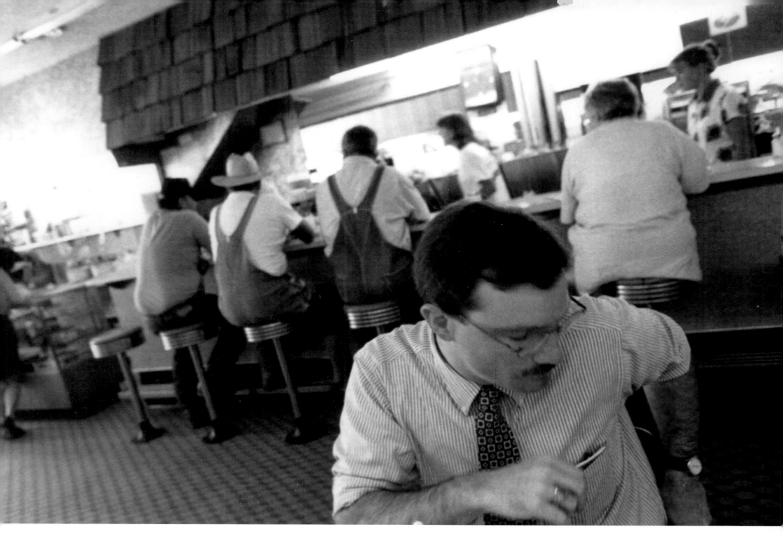

Lunch Break

After a quick bite at the Alsop and Graham Drug Store on the Courthouse Square in Fayette, Foster is ready to head back to the clinic to see afternoon patients. Howard County's agricultural economy is evident from the farmers in overalls at the lunch counter.

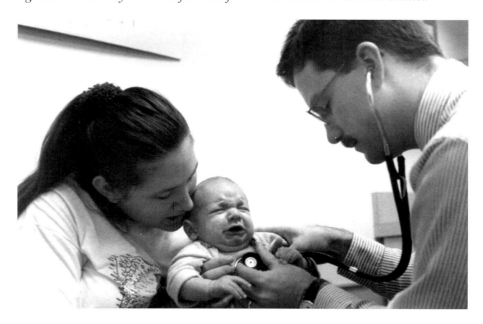

Well-Child Exam

Foster examines 2-month-old David Phipps, who seems less than happy about it. He is the first child of Wendy Phipps, left, and Randy Phipps, who works as a tobacco cutter near their Salisbury, Mo., home.

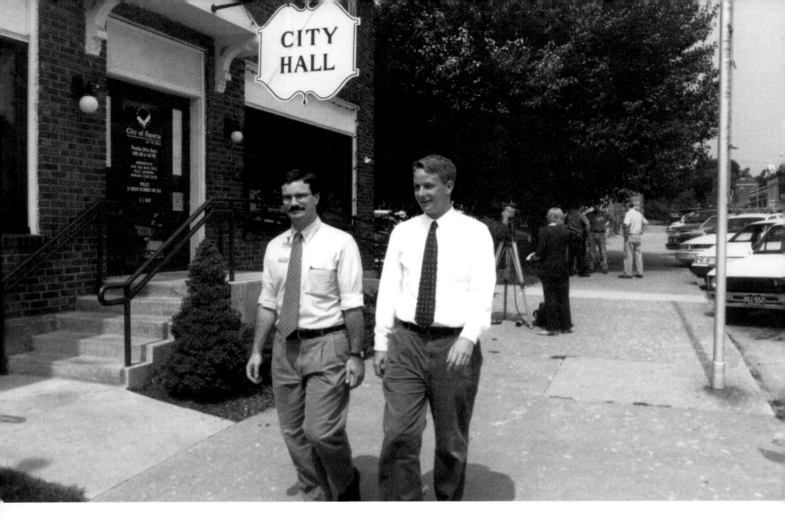

Downtown Fayette

*Foster, left, and Tom Sommers walk
past Fayette's City Hall, just off the
Courthouse Square (background).
Sommers, a fourth-year medical student
at Washington University in St. Louis,
was working with Foster for a month.
Fayette, a Central Missouri community
of 3,000, is home to historic Central
Methodist College.*

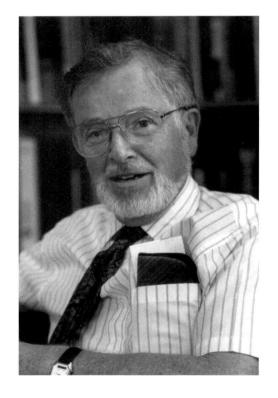

Medical Educator

*Jack Colwill, M.D., a nationally
known leader in family medicine
and primary care education, is the
longtime chairman of the
Department of Family and
Community Medicine at the
University of Missouri–Columbia
School of Medicine.*

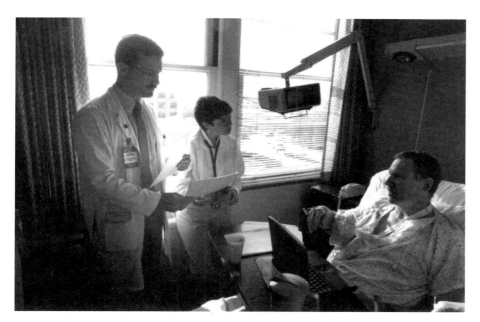

Doctor for a Patient

Foster and attending physician and faculty member Anne Fitzsimmons, M.D., making rounds at University Hospital, find Dr. Gilbert Youmans, a professor of English at MU, working at his portable computer. Youmans was hospitalized after experiencing irregular heart rhythms.

Case Consultation

Foster, right, and other residents and medical students listen as Fitzsimmons discusses Youman's electrocardiogram at University Hospital. Fitzsimmons also is medical director of the Green Meadows Family Practice Center in Columbia.

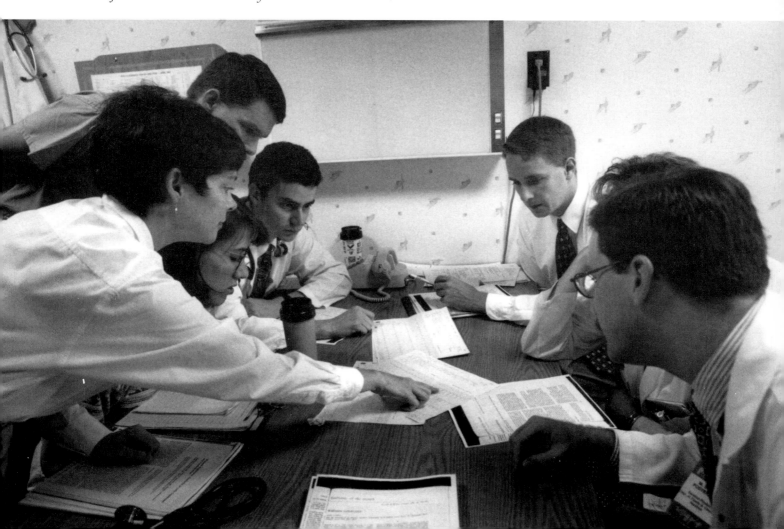

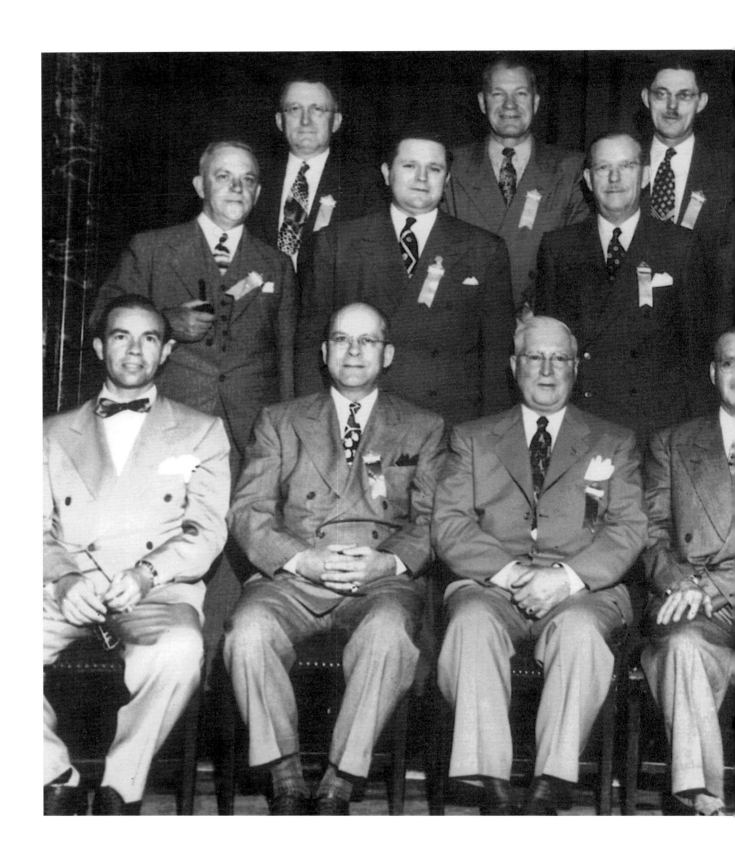

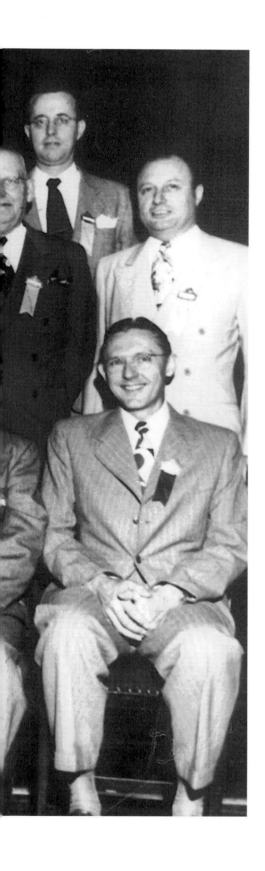

CHAPTER 5

Leading Generalism Into the 21st Century

"What if we establish an association to speak on behalf of general practitioners—what would happen then?" In 1947, when beleaguered general practitioners met in Atlantic City, N.J., to establish the American Academy of General Practice, the spirit that impelled them was the same spirit of adventure that moved Hippocrates, Semmelweis, Flexner, Willard and others to contribute significant advances to medical science or medical education. They questioned the status quo and came up with alternatives that worked.

Stanley Truman, M.D., of Oakland, Calif., was one of the sparkplugs who fired the AAGP's initial organizing efforts,

1947–49 National Officers
These were the national officers of the American Academy of General Practice one year after it was organized in 1947. Seated from left: Mac F. Cahal, J.D., executive secretary, Kansas City, Mo.; U.R. Bryner, M.D., treasurer, Salt Lake City; Paul A. Davis, M.D., president, Akron, Ohio; E.C. Texter, M.D., vice president, Detroit, and Stanley R. Truman, M.D., secretary, Oakland, Calif. Second row from left (all directors): G. Marchmont-Robinson, M.D., Chicago; H.T. Jackson, M.D., Fort Worth; R.C. McElvain, M.D., St. Louis; F.G. Benn, M.D., Minneapolis, and Lester D. Bibler, M.D., Indianapolis. Third row from left (all directors): Robert M. Lemmon, M.D., Akron, Ohio; Arch Walls, M.D., Detroit; J.P. Sanders, M.D., Shreveport, La., and D.G. Miller Jr., M.D., Morgantown, Ky. (Archives for Family Practice–AAFP Foundation.)

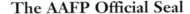

The AAFP Official Seal

The AAFP seal is rich in symbolism. The circle that forms the basis of the seal stands for "eternity and unity." The laurel branch at left symbolizes "honor, valor and victory." The oak leaves at right signify "divine knowledge." The ax or mace, capable of breaking through the strongest armor, represents "strength." In Greek, it stands for "the power of light over darkness." In Egyptian, the mace signifies "clever one" and "the cleaver of the way." The staff encircled by the serpent represents "healing" and "the renewing power of life." It is the traditional symbol of medicine, not to be confused with the Caduceus (a double-winged staff), which is the insignia of the military medical corps. (Archives for Family Practice–AAFP Foundation.)

serving as its first secretary and later as its president. He wrote the first chronicle of the Academy's early history. The first president, elected at the seminal meeting in Atlantic City, was Paul A. Davis, M.D., of Akron, Ohio.

Officers of the fledgling Academy found an executive secretary in Mac Cahal, J.D., previously chief executive officer and general counsel for the American College of Radiology, which he helped start 10 years earlier.

Truman described Cahal as "formerly a newspaper man, master organizer, a perfect writer and a smooth personality." He proved to be an excellent choice. Serving until 1971, Cahal said later in an interview that his biggest contribution to the Academy was "to give prestige and dignity to the general practitioners. They had been discriminated against for years, and were considered nobodies among medical organizations."

The Academy's national headquarters was established in 1948 in Kansas City, Mo. (still the Academy's hometown). The first Congress of Delegates, the Academy's highest policy-making body, was convened that same year in Chicago. The first Annual Scientific Assembly, the Academy's largest continuing medical education meeting for members, was held in Cincinnati in 1949.

Using his journalism background, Cahal started *GP* magazine in 1950, when Academy membership had swelled to 10,000. He hired experts in design and printing, and selected only the best writers for the assigned articles. Advertising was relegated to the back pages. *GP's* use of editorial color was a first in medical journalism. Quickly, the publication (now *American Family Physician*) became known as one of the best medical journals in the nation.

The AAGP grew steadily as GPs recognized its effectiveness in reprofessionalizing general practice and enhancing the public's recognition of their important role in medicine. They were proud of the Academy's requirement that they complete 150 hours of continuing medical education every three years in order to remain members.

In 1965, after years of intensive debate, the Academy's Congress of Delegates voted to seek establishment of family practice as a new medical "specialty in breadth." In 1967, the Society of Teachers of Family Medicine was founded to aid in the development of training programs for the specialty-to-be, to provide a discussion forum for those involved in family health care and to expand the body of knowledge of family medicine. Academy member Lynn Carmichael, M.D., of the University of Miami was its original organizer and first president; the society's headquarters moved to Kansas City in 1972.

The efforts of the Academy's leaders and others finally succeeded in 1969, when the independent American Board of Family Practice was approved and the new specialty born. The board's founding executive secretary was Academy member Nicholas J. Pisacano, M.D., a faculty member at the University of Kentucky in Lexington, still the board's headquarters city. Two years later, the AAGP changed its name to the American Academy of Family Physicians (AAFP).

From its meager beginnings—the AAGP's net worth in May of 1948 was $74,000—the Academy has grown into a multimillion-dollar organization with nearly 270 employees. In the 1995–96 fiscal year, the AAFP spent more than $45 million providing services, programs and publications for its more than 80,000 members. About 45,000 of those are "active" members, mostly practicing physicians and family medicine teachers. Another 28,000 are medical students interested in family practice, and family practice residents.

The AAFP is governed by the Congress of Delegates, composed of two representatives each from chapters in the 50 states, District of Columbia, Puerto Rico, the Virgin Islands, Guam and the uniformed services. The Congress also includes two delegates each for these AAFP constituencies: medical students, family practice residents, women, minorities and new physicians (those in practice seven or fewer years). Between meetings of the Congress, the AAFP Board of Directors establishes policies and defines principles, subject to approval by the next Congress.

Held right after each meeting of the Congress of Delegates is the Annual Scientific Assembly, one of the premier continuing medical education meetings in the nation. It regularly draws about 17,000 physicians, guests, exhibitors and others.

In addition to *American Family Physician (AFP)*, the Academy publishes *Family Practice Management* journal, as well as several news publications for its members and leaders. The journals' advertising sales offices are in New Jersey, and *AFP's* medical editing office is at Georgetown University Medical Center in Washington, D.C.

The work of the Academy is carried out by the elected officers and directors, the professional staff and members who volunteer on nine standing commissions and more than eight committees. Besides the headquarters in

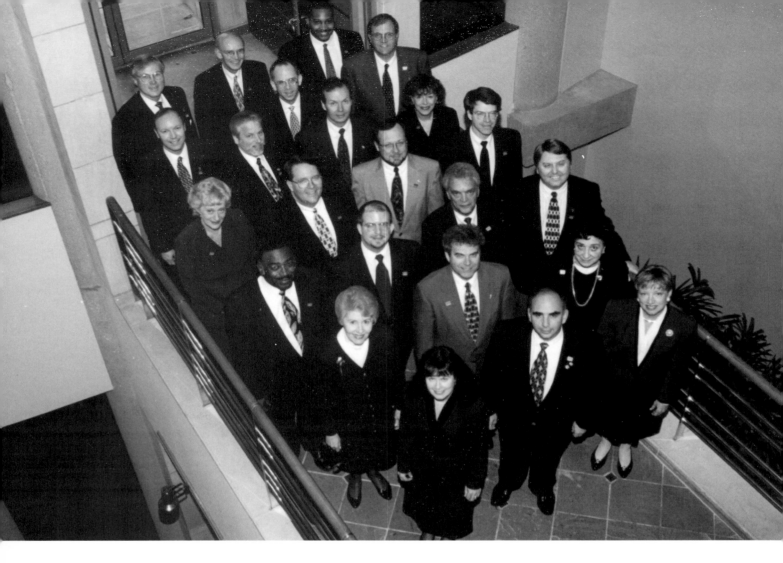

1996-97 AAFP Board and Senior Staff

The AAFP's 1996–97 Board of Directors and senior staff reflect the growing diversity of the Academy's membership.

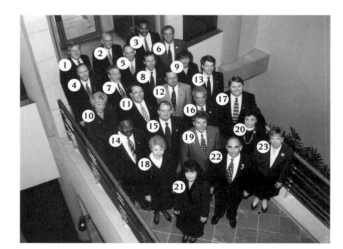

1. Lanny Copeland, M.D., Moultrie, Ga., director
2. Robert Graham, M.D., Kansas City, Mo., executive vice president
3. Jimmie Smith Jr., M.D., Albany, Ga., resident director
4. Bruce Bagley, M.D., Latham, N.Y., director
5. Douglas E. Henley, M.D., Fayetteville, N.C., Board chair
6. Philip D. Briggs, M.D., Santa Fe, N.M., director
7. Ronald E. Christensen, M.D., Anchorage, Alaska, director
8. Joseph E. Scherger, M.D., M.P.H., San Diego, director
9. Clayton R. Hasser, Kansas City, Mo., vice president for publications and communications
10. Susan Black, M.D., Lowell, Mass., vice president
11. Michael O. Fleming, M.D., Shreveport, La., vice speaker
12. David L. Massanari, M.D., Sanford, Maine, director
13. David M. West, M.D., Grand Junction, Colo., director
14. Melvin D. Gerald, M.D., M.P.H., Washington, director
15. David Hutcheson-Tipton, Denver, student director
16. R. Michael Miller, J.D., Kansas City, Mo., deputy executive vice president
17. Richard G. Roberts, M.D., J.D., Madison, Wis., speaker
18. JoAnn Rockufeler, Kansas City, Mo., executive assistant
19. Patrick B. Harr, M.D., Maryville, Mo., president
20. Rose Mary Hatem Bonsack, M.D., Aberdeen, Md., director
21. Rosemarie Sweeney, Washington, vice president for socioeconomic affairs and policy analysis
22. Neil H. Brooks, M.D., Rockville, Conn., president-elect
23. Mickey Schaefer, Kansas City, Mo., vice president for administration; meetings and conventions; membership

(Not pictured: Daniel J. Ostergaard, M.D., Kansas City, Mo., vice president for education and scientific affairs)

Kansas City, AAFP maintains a legislative and public policy office in Washington, D.C., and a clinical policy analysis office at the University of Washington in Seattle.

The Academy works with the United States Congress, state legislators, other medical societies, national media, medical academia and business leaders to address a broad range of health-care issues. Examples include rural medicine, the cost and quality of care in evolving health-care delivery systems, Medicare and Medicaid reform, clinical guidelines development and access to care for America's uninsured and underinsured. Another key Academy function is to enhance the image of family practice and the public's respect for family physicians.

The AAFP promotes medical student interest in family practice and offers advice and support to the more than 450 residency programs across the nation.

It also actively promotes family physician education in other countries. It is an organizational member of the World Organization of Family Doctors (known as WONCA) and has served as a networking entity for AAFP members in their individual humanitarian efforts.

For four years, the Academy has partnered with Heart to Heart International and the AAFP Foundation in the Physicians With Heart program, which has airlifted more than $27 million worth of donated pharmaceuticals, supplies and equipment to former Soviet republics that desperately need the help.

Robert Graham, M.D., the AAFP's current executive vice president, predicts that the Academy and family practice will continue to play a major role in American health care. "Family physicians will become more in demand and more clearly a centerpoint of an efficiently operating health-care system," he says. He discounts predictions that patients of the future will become "their own doctors with little diagnostic computers."

"I think people will still want the human interface with someone who is more knowledgeable than they about how the body works, what the risk factors are and how to take care of life's little problems that may be life's big problems in disguise," he says.

As it was in the past, the AAFP's role into the 21st century will be intertwined with those of the other family practice organizations. For without the Academy, the role of the generalist in medicine likely would have withered into extinction—but without the American Board of Family Practice, the Academy might not have grown into the powerhouse it is today. And without the Society of Teachers of Family Medicine and other, more recent academic family medicine organizations, there might not have been a teacher corps sufficient to train today's modern family physicians.

These organizations in the "family of family practice" will continue to work together to ensure that tomorrow, there will be enough well-trained family physicians to care for America.

Bibliography

General References
AAFP Historical Perspectives. Mac F. Cahal, J.D., Stanley R. Truman, M.D., Nicholas Pisacano, M.D., and B. Leslie Huffman, M.D. A video series of the American Academy of Family Physicians.
Cahal, Mac F. *A Twentieth Century Renaissance in American Medicine.* Paper presented before the first annual meeting of the Congress of Delegates of the American Academy of General Practice, Chicago, June 21, 1948.
The Changing Pattern of Medical Practice and a New Specialty of Family Medicine. A collection of quotations from medical practitioners and educators. American Academy of General Practice. Kansas City, 1969.
The Graduate Education of Physicians. Chicago: Report of the Citizens Commission on Graduate Medical Education, commissioned by the American Medical Association, 1966.
Health Is a Community Affair. Cambridge, Mass.: Harvard University Press, Report of the National Commission on Community Health Services, sponsored by the American Public Health Association and National Health Council, 1966.
A Historical Sketch of Family Practice. Kansas City: American Academy of Family Physicians, 1976.
Meeting the Challenge of Family Practice. Chicago: Report of the Ad Hoc Committee on Education for Family Practice of the Council on Medical Education, American Medical Association, 1966.

Books
Bryan, James E. *The Role of the Family Physician in America's Developing Medical Care Program.* St. Louis: The Family Health Foundation of America, 1968.
Carmichael, Ann G., and Ratzan, Richard M. *Medicine: A Treasury of Art and Literature.* New York: Hugh Lauter Leven Associates, Inc., 1991.
Clark, Howard C., M.D. *A History of the Sedgwick County, Kansas, Medical Society.*
Facts About Family Practice. Kansas City: American Academy of Family Physicians, 1996.
Family Practice: Creation of a Specialty. Kansas City: American Academy of Family Physicians, 1980.
Geyman, John P. *Family Practice: Foundation of Changing Health Care.* New York: Appleton-Century-Crofts, 1980.
Hahn, Mary L., and Reilly, Blanche. *Bollinger County: 1851–1976.* Marceline, Mo.: Walsworth Publishing Co., 1977.
History of Southeast Missouri. Chicago: The Goodspeed Publishing Co., 1888.
History of Wright County, Minnesota. Buffalo: 1914.
Lyons, Albert S., and Petrucelli, R. Joseph II. *Medicine: An Illustrated History.* New York: Harry N. Abrams, Inc., 1978.
Nuland, Sherwin B. *Doctors: The Biography of Medicine.* New York: Vintage Books, 1988.
The Physician. LIFE Science Library. Time, Inc., 1967.
Richards, Dickinson W., M.D. "Hippocrates and History: The Arrogance of Humanism," *In Search of the Modern Hippocrates* (Edited by Roger J. Bulger, M.D.) Iowa City: University of Iowa Press, 1987.
Stephens, G. Gayle, M.D. *The Intellectual Basis of Family Practice.* Tucson, Ariz.: Winter Publishing Company, Inc., 1982.
Truman, Stanley R. *The History of the Founding of the American Academy of General Practice.* St. Louis: Warren H. Green, Inc., 1969.
Williams, Charles Hamilton. *I Remember the Ozarks.* (Edited by Nelda Mayfield Wilkinson.) Marble Hill, Mo.: Stewart Printing & Publishing Co., 1995.
The World Book Encyclopedia. Chicago: World Book, Inc., 1988.

Periodicals
"The Academy's Story: 1947–1972." *AAFP Daily News,* September 1972.
Adams, David P. "Evolution of the Specialty of Family Practice." Jacksonville: *Journal of the Florida Medical Association,* March 1989.
Canfield, Phillip R. "Family Medicine: An Historical Perspective." *Journal of Medical Education,* 1976.
"Country Doctor Lloyd McCaskill." *TODAY'S HEALTH.* American Medical Association, 1961.
Garrison, Richard L. "The Five Generations of American Medical Revolutions." *The Journal of Family Practice,* March 1995.
Hunt, Vincent R. "The Unifying Principles of Family Medicine: A Historical Perspective." Providence: *Rhode Island Medicine,* July 1993.
McKee, Denise, and Chappel, John N. "Spirituality and Medical Practice." *The Journal of Family Practice,* August 1992.
Titone, Julie. "Medicine Man." *American Medical News,* June 1990.
Wilson, Vernon. "Specialist in Family Practice—Prototype of a Doctor." Kansas City: *GP,* August 1969.

Index

A

AAFP Board of Directors, 121
AAFP Foundation, 1, 123
AAFP's 1996–97 Board of Directors, 122
ABC Health, 88
Aberdeen, Md., 122
Ad Hoc Committee on Education for Family Practice, 34
Aegean Sea, 15
African-American, 61
AIDS, 19, 98
Akron, Ohio, 119, 120
Alabama, 9, 78, 79, 80, 81, 83
Alaska, 43, 51, 53, 122
Alaska and Polar Regions Department, 43
Albany, Ga., 122
Albrecht, C. Earl, 43
Albrecht, Margie, 43
alcohol, 51, 91
Alexander, Cole, 70
Allegheny University of the Health Sciences, 30, 42
Alsop and Graham Drug Store, 115
Alspaugh, Elena, 94
Alspaugh, Emil Benjamin, 94
Alspaugh, Kevin, 94
AMA Council on Medical Education, 34
Amarillo, Texas, 104
American Academy of Family Physicians, 7, 9, 35, 57, 121
American Academy of Family Physicians Foundation, 1, 7, 9, 35
American Academy of General Practice, 7, 33, 34, 35, 119
American Board of Family Practice, 34, 121, 123
American College of Radiology, 120
American College of Surgeons, 31
American Family Physician, 120, 121
American Gothic, 99
American Indians, 9, 15, 45, 106
American Medical Association, 33
American Public Health Association, 34
American Red Cross, 9, 40
American Women's Hospital Service, 42
anatomy, 17
Anchorage, Alaska, 43, 122
Annandale, Minn., 7, 37, 39
Annette Island Indian Reserve, 53
Annual Scientific Assembly, 120, 121
antibiotics, 19
Appalachia, 93
Archives and Special Collections on Women in Medicine, 30, 42
Archives for Family Practice, 10, 119, 120
Arizona, 9, 53, 73, 76, 104
Arizona House, 76
Arizona Senate, 76
Arizona State University, 53
Arizonans Concerned About Smoking, 9, 73
Arkansas, 10, 32, 89
Arlington, Vt., 101
Arms, Leslie, 112
Art Resource, dust jacket back flap
aseptic surgery, 19, 27

Association of American Indian Physicians, 55
Atlanta, Ga., 61
Atlantic City, N.J., 7, 119, 120
Augsburg College, 73
Augsburger, Bryan, 60
Augsburger, Julie, 60
Augsburger, Kade, 60
Aultman, Oliver E., 29

B

Bagley, Bruce, 122
Bailey, N.C., 106
Baines, Catherine, 53, 55
Baines, David R., 9, 50, 51, 52, 53, 54, 55
Ballard, Linda, 94
Balsam Grove, N.C., 46
Baltimore, Md., 27
Bathgate Health Center, 87
Battle of the Bulge, 67, 106
Beamont (Texas) Enterprise, 128
Beijing, China, 73
Benn, F.G., 119
Bentley Historical Library, 18, 31, 32
Beth Israel Medical Center, 88
Bethesda, Md., 10, 14, 15, 16, 25, 40, 61
Bibler, Lester D., 119
Binder, Paula Haas, 10
Black, Susan, 122
Blackmon, Erick, 79
Blaine, Jim, 72
Bloodworth-Thomason, Linda, 128
Blue Ridge Mountains, 47
Bodily, Sherri, 95
Bollinger County, Mo., 4
Bonsack, Rose Mary Hatem, 122
Bosnia, 65
Boston, Mass., 60
Boston's Lying In Hospital, 23
Bradenton, Fla., 43
Bradley, Florence, 68
Bradley, Jennifer, 68
Brandon Hospital, 41
Brandon, Walter L., 41
Bremerton, Wash., Naval Hospital, 63
Briggs, Philip D., 122
Bronx-Lebanon Hospital, 84, 86, 88
Brooks, Neil H., 122
Broseley, Mo., 41
Brown University, 61
Bruce Roberts Collection, 44, 45, 46, 47, 48, 106
Bryner, U.R., 119
bubonic plague, 17
Burke, Grafton, 43
Burke, Michael, 50
Busse, John, 83
Butler County: A Pictorial History, 128
Butler County, Mo., 24

C

Cable, Dennis, 57
caduceus, 120
Cahal, Mac F., 119, 120
California, 50, 87, 97, 119, 122
Callaway Clinic, 109
Callaway Community Hospital, 110
Callaway Physicians, 110
Calman, Neil R., 9, 84, 85, 86, 87
Camden, Ala., 80, 81

Campbell County, Tenn., 89
Canadian, 27
cancer, 19
Cannon, Blaine, 46, 47, 48
Capitol building, 25
Carmichael, Lynn, 121
Carnegie Foundation, 29
Carter, D.E., Mrs., 107
Carter, Darrell, 107
Casler, Shirley, Sister, 81, 83
Catholic, 57, 83
Cedar Rapids Museum of Art, 99
Center for American History, The, 44, 45, 46, 47, 48, 106
Central America, 91
Central Dispensary and Emergency Hospital, 25
Central Methodist College, 116
Chandler, Ariz., 104
Chandler, Kevin, 114
Chaney, Matt, 128
Charity Hospital of Louisiana, 75
Chartran, T., 14
Cheyenne, Wyo., 53
Chicago, Ill., 119, 120
Chicago Medical School, 61
Chicago Tribune, 103
childbed fever, 19
Christensen, Ronald E., 122
Christmas, 81, 97
Churches of Christ, 89
CIA, 57
CIGNA, 77
CIGNA Healthplan's Stapley Health Care Center, 73
Cincinnati, Ohio, 120
circulation, 17
Citizens Commission on Graduate Medical Education, 34
Clairfield, Tenn., 89
Coeur d'Alene Tribe, 55
Coeur d'Alene Indian Reservation, 9, 51
Coeur d'Alene River, 52
Colorado, 29, 122
Colorado Historical Society, 29
Columbia, Mo., 104, 117
Colwill, Jack, 10, 113, 116
Congress of Delegates, 120, 121
Connecticut, 13, 15, 27, 122
Cook, Roseanne, Sister, 9, 78, 79, 80, 81, 82, 83
Copeland, Lanny, 122
Corral, Silvia, 9, 94, 95, 96, 97, 98
Cos, 15
Country Doctor Museum, 106
Crane, Jack, 52
Crane, Lynda, 52
Crossnore, N.C., 102
Crotona Park, 87
Crump, J. W., 104
Cumberland Mountains, 92
Curran, Angela, 10
Cyprus, 57

D

D-Day, 67
Daily American Republic, 128
Davis, Paul A., 119, 120
Denver, Colo., 122
Destefano, Mayra, 87
Detroit, Mich., 119
diabetes, 51, 98

District of Columbia, 121
Doctor, The, endsheets, dust jacket back flap
Doctors: The Biography of Medicine, 15
Dominican Republic, 59
Dorsey, J. G., 11
drug problems, 91, 94, 95
Dublin, Ga., 35
Duke University Medical Center, 57

E

East Tennessee, 9
Edwards, Merdal, 25
Egyptians, 15, 120
Ekern, H.P. "Pete," 107
Elam, Jim R., 10, 113, 114
Elkland, Mo., 106
Epp, Mary Ann, 77
ether, 19, 112
Europe, 17, 106

F

Fairbanks, Eunice, 75, 77
Fairbanks, Leland L., 9, 73, 74, 75, 76, 77
Family Doctor, 99
Family Practice Management, 121
Farrington, F.B., 25
Fathers of St. Edmund, 83
Faulkner, Ritter, 88
Fayette, Mo., 110, 114, 115, 116
Fayette, Mo., Medical Clinic, 110, 114
Fayetteville, N.C., 122
Fildes, Luke, Sir, dust jacket back flap
Fitzsimmons, Anne, 117
Flagler College, 60
Flash-Lighters of Minneappolis, 20
Fleming, Michael O., 122
Flexner, Abraham, 29, 119
Florida, 9, 41, 43, 56, 57, 58, 59, 60, 61, 81, 121
Florida State Archives, 41
Flowers, Audrey, 50
Folsom Report, 34
Formby, Thomas, 89, 93
Fort Crook, Neb., Army Hospital, 106
Fort Porter, N.Y., 9
Fort Worth, 119
4th Street Clinic, 95, 97, 98
Foster, Shane, 10, 114, 115, 116, 117
Fowler, Cleta, 57
France, 40, 67
Francis A. Countway Library of Medicine, 23
Francis, Iva, 66
Frontier Nursing Service, 42
Ft. Yukon, Alaska, 43
Fulton, Mo., 109, 110, 112, 114

G

Galen, 17
Galluzzo, Chester, 76, 77
Galluzzo, Geraldine, 76, 77
Garden City, Kan., 29
Gaw, Steve, 72
Generalist Physician Initiative, 113
Genuine Christianity, 92
George, Earlie, 66
Georgetown University Medical Center, 121
Georgia, 35, 61, 63, 122

Georgia Department of Archives and
History, 35
Gerald, Melvin D., 122
German, 19, 27, 67
GI Bill, 31
Glaxo Wellcome Inc., 1
GP, 120
Grace Busse Clinic, 81
Graham, Robert, 122, 123
Grand Coulee Dam, 50
Grand Junction, Colo., 122
Gray, R. E., 29
Great Depression, 73
Greek, 15, 17, 120
Green Meadows Family Practice
Center, 110, 117
Greene County Medical Society, 72
Greentop, Mo., 25
Guam, 121
Guantanamo Bay, Cuba, 63

H
Haiti, 61, 63, 65
Hampton, Hiram, 41
Handbook of Early American Art, 1
Hangman Creek, 55
Harbison, Grant, 50
Harlow, Bernadette, 62
Harlow, Noah, 62
Harlow, Philip, 62
Harper's Weekly, 15, 16
Harr, Patrick B., 7, 122
Harris, Clifford, 77
Harrison, Terry, 112
Hartman, Anne, 60
Hartman, Cleta, 60
Hartman, Heidi, 60
Hartman, John R., 9, 56, 57, 58, 59,
60
Hartman, Karen, 60
Harvard Medical School, 23
Harvard Report, 34
Harvey Cushing/John Hay Whitney
Medical Library, 13, 27
Harvey, Ill., 105
Harvey, William, 17
Hasser, Clayton R., 122
Heart to Heart International, 123
heart disease, 19
Henley, Douglas E., 122
Hensley, Glenn, 107
Hernet, Rosemarie, 107
Hickory, N.C., 114
Hippocrates, 13, 15, 17, 19, 35, 119
Hispanic, 85
HIV, 63, 91
HMO, 77
Holliday, Milton J., 24
Holy Redeemer Catholic Church, 56,
59
homicide, 51
Honduras, 84
hookworm, 40
Hosmer, Craig, 72
Howard County, Mo., 115
Hudson Stuck Memorial Hospital, 43
Huff, Bonnie, 90
Huff, Bryana Elizabeth, 90
Hunter, Joe, 105
Hurricane Opal, 83
Hutcheson-Tipton, David, 122
hypertension, 51

I
Idaho, 9, 51, 52, 53, 55
Idaho Department of Health, 52
Idaho Panhandle, 51
Illinois, 61, 85, 87, 89, 103, 105, 119,
120
Imhotep, 15
immunology, 17
Indian Health Service, 53, 73
Indian Mountain, 89
Indian Mountain Clinic, 89, 92
Indiana, 67, 119
Indiana University, 67
Indianapolis, Ind., 67, 119
Institute for Urban Family Health, 9,
84, 85, 87
Institute of Medicine, 113
International Union for Circumpolar
Health, 43
Iowa, 18, 22, 99

J
Jackson, H.T., 119
Jackson, Mo., 111
Jacksonville, Fla., Naval Hospital, 61
Japan, 61
Jellico Community Hospital, 90, 91
Jellico, Tenn., 9, 89, 92
Jenner, Edward, 17
Jewish, 85
John F. Kennedy Memorial Medical
Center, 75
John Paul Jones Hospital, 81
johnboat, 42
Johns Hopkins, 27, 29
Jones, Joey, 90

K
Kansas, 11, 29
Kansas City, Mo., 67, 119, 120, 121,
122, 123
Kansas City, Mo., General Hospital,
67
Kansas State Historical Society, 29
Kentucky, 40, 42, 89, 119, 121
Keokuk Medical College, 11
Ketchikan, Alaska, 53
Kings Bay, Ga., 63
Kissimmee, Fla., 9, 56, 57, 59
Kneibert, Fred L., 4
Knoxville, 89
Koch, Robert, 19
Koshney, Paul, 50
Krohn, Eugene, 21

L
Laatsch, Robert H., 41
*Laennec Listening with His Ear Against
the Chest of a Patient at Necker
Hospital*, 14
Laennec, Rene, 17, 20
Lamons, Matthew, 113
Lange, Dorothea, 104
Latham, N.Y., 122
Laurel Fork-Clear Fork Health
Centers, 89
Lemmon, Robert M., 119
Lewis, Evelyn, 10, 61, 62, 63, 64, 65
Li, Kenneth C., 4
Liberia, 73, 75
Lindberg Collection, The, 43
Lister, Joseph, 19
Little Rock, Ark., 32
liver cirrhosis, 51

London, dust jacket back flap
Long, Crawford, 19
Louisiana, 75, 119, 122
Lowell, Mass., 122
Lucy Lee Healthcare System, 105
Lymon, Margaret, 78

M
Macdonnell, Ann Martin, 67, 70
Macdonnell, C.R., 66, 68, 69, 103,
106
Macdonnell, Tommy, 9, 66, 67, 68,
69, 70, 71, 72, 103, 106, 107
Madison, Wis., 122
Maine, 122
Malakooti, Mark, 64
Malakooti, Nicola, 64
Malakooti, Susan, 64
malaria, 63
Manhattan, 84, 86, 88
Manhattan's Union Square, 87
Marble Hill, Mo., 4, 20
Marchmont-Robinson, G., 119
Marnell, Paul, Mrs., 107
Marshfield, Mo., 9, 67, 69, 71, 103
Martinez, Juan, 84
Maryland, 10, 15, 16, 20, 23, 25, 27,
29, 40, 61, 122
Maryville, Mo., 122
Massachusetts, 23, 34, 60, 122
Massanari, David L., 122
Matanuska Valley, 43
Maxton, 44
Mayfield, William Henderson, 4
Mayo (Clinic) Medical School, 53
McCall's, 83
McCaskill, Lloyd, 44, 45
McClain, Monroe D., 32
McClain, Monroe D., Jr., 32
McElvain, R.C., 119
McLeod, Mary, 55
McPheeters, J. W., 105
McRay, Anna, 89, 93
McRay, David, 9, 88, 89, 90, 91, 93
McRay, Joan, 89, 93
McRay, Jonathan, 89, 93
McRay, Michael, 89, 93
measles, 63, 107
Medicaid, 88, 89, 123
Medicare, 33, 123
Meharry Medical College, 61
Mesa, Ariz., 9, 73
Methodist, 51
Mexico, 97
Mexico, Mo., 107
Michigan, 18, 31, 32, 119
microscope, 20
Middle Ages, 17
Middle East, 65
Miller, D.G., Jr., 119
Miller, R. Michael, 122
Millis Commission, 34
Milwaukee, 107
Milwaukee Journal, 107
Minneapolis, Minn., 37, 73, 105, 119
Minneapolis Star, 128
Minneapolis Star–Journal–Tribune, 7,
37
Minnesota, 7, 14, 37, 39, 53, 73, 104,
105, 119
Minnesota Historical Society, 7, 20,
37, 104, 105
Missouri, 1, 4, 8, 9, 10, 11, 14, 24, 25,
41, 67, 69, 71, 72, 81, 103, 104,

105, 106, 107, 109, 110, 111, 112,
114, 115, 116, 117, 119, 120, 121,
122, 123, 128
Missouri Farmer, The, 107
Missouri House of Representatives,
69
Missouri State Archives, 25
Modesto, Calif., 50
Montauk, N.Y., 23
Montefiore Medical Center, 87
Montessori school, 95
Montgomery, Ala., 79
Morgantown, Ky., 119
Morrisania Hospital, 87
Morrisette, Jesse, 78, 79, 80, 81
Motorola Company, 57
Moultrie, Ga., 122

N
Nashville, Tenn., 61, 89
National Academy of Sciences, 113
National Archives, 104
National Commission on Community
Health Services, 34
National Health Council, 34
National Health Service Corps, 89
National Library of Medicine, 14, 15,
16, 23, 25, 40
Native Americans, 51, 53, 54, 55
Nazi, 71, 106
Nearing, Katie, 58
Nebraska, 106
Nebraska State Historical Society,
106
Neptune Elementary School, 58
New Jersey, 7, 85, 119, 120, 121
New Mexico, 104, 122
New Orleans, La., 75
New York, 9, 23, 101, 122
New York City, 9, 15, 16, 84, 85, 86,
87, 88, dust jacket back flap
New York State Academy of Family
Physicians, 88
Newcomb, Kate, 103
Newell, Josephine E., 106
Nigeria, 73
Nigerian, 73, 75
Nikon, 11
Norfolk, Va., 75
Norman Rockwell Family Trust, 101
Norman Rockwell Museum at
Stockbridge, The, 101
Norman Rockwell Visits a Family Doctor,
100, 101
Normandy Invasion, 67
North Bronx, N.Y., 87
North Carolina, 44, 57, 102, 114, 122
North Carolina Division of Archives
and History, 102
Northwestern University, 89
Nuland, Sherwin B., 15, 17

O
Oakland, Calif., 119
obesity, 51
Ohio, 119, 120
Okinawa, Japan, 63
Oklahoma, 113
Oregon, 106
Osler, William, Sir, 27
Ostergaard, Daniel J., 122
Ozark Mountains, 9, 20, 69, 103, 128

P

Palmer, Alaska, 43
Paré, Ambroise, 17
Parkchester, 87
Pasteur, Louis, 19, 20
pathology, 19
Pavelin, Andrew, 103
Peabody, George, 89
Pennsylvania Hospital, 30
Pensacola Naval Air Station Hospital, 57
Perkins, Mildred, 24
Pettitt, Marguaret, 68
Philadelphia, Pa., 30, 102
Phipps, David, 115
Phipps, Randy, 115
Phipps, Wendy, 115
Phoenix, Ariz., 53
Physicians With Heart, 123
Picha, Eunice, 73
Pine Apple, Ala., 78, 81
Pine Mountain, 9, 89, 92
Pioneer Park, 98
Pisacano, Nicholas J., 121
polio, 19, 105, 106, 107
Poplar Bluff, Mo., 41, 105, 128
Porter, John, dust jacket back flap
Poughkeepsie, N.Y., 101
Pratt, Allan, 60
Prince George County, Va., 75
Principles and Practices of Medicine, 27
Puerto Rico, 121

R

Racinowski, Donald, 114
radium, 19
Reed, C.C., 32
Reeds, Willie, 78, 79, 81
Regionalism, 99
Renaissance, 17
Residency Review Committee for Family Practice, 35
Rhode Island, 61
Richardson, Ethel, 88
Richardson, Mitchael, 88
Richardson, Seth, 88
Rickey, J.K., 22
Ridgway, Alfred M., 7, 37, 38, 39
Rio Grande neighborhood, 97
Robb, Ann, 73
Robert Wood Johnson Foundation, 113
Roberts, Bruce, 44, 46
Roberts, Richard G., 122
Robledo, Antonia, 74
Rochester, Minn., 53
Rockufeler, JoAnn, 122
Rockville, Conn., 122
Rockwell, Norman, 10, 100, 101
Rockwell, Thomas, 10, 101
Rohlf, W.A., 18
Roman Catholic, 9, 56, 79, 80
Roman Empire, 17
Roper, Helen, 70
Rush University, 87
Russell, George A., 100, 101
Rutgers Medical School, 85

S

Sainz, Irene, 74
Saipan, 57
Salisbury, Mo., 115
Salk, 106, 107

Salt Lake City, Utah, 9, 95, 96, 119
Salt Lake City-County Health Department, 97
Salt Lake Regional Health Center, 97, 98
San Diego, Calif., 122
Sanders, J.P., 119
Sanders, Kathy Wolpers, 10
Sanford, Maine, 122
Santa Barbara, Calif., 97
Santa Fe., N.M., 122
Saskatchewan, 54, 55
Saturday Evening Post, 101
Schabbing, Mark B., 10, 109, 111, 112
Schaefer, Mickey, 122
Scherger, Joseph E., 122
Schneiderheinze, Nancy, 10
Searcy, Ark., 89
Searle, 55
Seattle, Wash., 40, 123
Semmelweis, Ignaz, 19, 119
Seventh Day Adventist Church, 91
Shearon, Dolores, 10
Shreveport, La., 119, 122
Sick Woman in Bellevue Hospital, New York, Overrun by Rats, The, 15
Sider, Ronald J., 92
Sidney Hillman Family Practice Center, 86, 87
SiJohn, Merle, 55
Silver Star Medal, 67
Sioux, 53
Sisters of St. Joseph of Carondelet, 79
Slater, Kathryn Hunter, 105
Sloop, Eustace, 102
Sloop, Mary Martin, 102
smallpox, 17
Smith, Jimmie, Jr., 122
Smither, William J., 11
Society of Teachers of Family Medicine, 121, 123
Somalia, 65
Sommers, Tom, 116
South Alabama, 79, 83
South Bronx, N.Y., 86, 87
South Carolina, 42
South Dakota, 53
South-Paul, Jeannette, 63
Southeast Alaska, 51
Southern California, 87
Soviet Union, 61
Spanish influenza, 9, 40
Spanish-American War, 23
Spartanburg, S.C., 42
Spelman College, 61
Springfield, Mo., 69, 72
St. Augustine, Fla., 60
St. Joseph's Catholic Church, 80
St. Louis, Mo., 81, 116, 119
St. Louis College of Physicians and Surgeons, 4
St. Louis Medical College, 20
St. Louis University, 25
St. Maries, Idaho, 51, 52, 53
St. Paul, Minn., 20, 104
Stallworth, Melvin, 82
Stanard, John R., 11, 128
Stanard, Michael J., 128
Stanard, Roberts V., 105
Stanard, Vida Loberg, 10, 128
Stanford University, 97
State Historical Society of Iowa, 18, 22

State Historical Society of Missouri, dust jacket back flap, 1
State Historical Society of Wisconsin, 21, 103, 117
State University of Iowa, 18
Steele, Blaine, 86
stethoscope, 14, 17, 31
Stevermer, James, 109
suicide, 51
sulfa drugs, 19
Sweeney, Rosemarie, 122

T

Talley, William, 20
Tampa, Fla., 61
Tate Gallery, dust jacket back flap
Taylor, H. Longstreet, 20
Teasdale, Joe, 70
Tenncare, 89
Tennessee, 9, 61, 89, 90, 91, 92
Tennessee Academy of Family Physicians, 89
Tennessee River, 93
Teutonic, 17
Texas, 44, 45, 46, 47, 48, 104, 106, 119
Texter, E.C., 119
Thompson, William C., 35
Tlingit Tribe, 51, 54
Travelers Aid Society, 98
Treloar, Harry, 53
Trinidad, Colo., 29
Truman, Harry S, 41
Truman, Stanley R., 119
Trumble, Marilyn, 68
Tsimshian Tribe, 51
tuberculosis, 14, 51, 63, 98
Tulsa, Okla., 113
Turley, Stan, 76
Turner, Harriet Y., 99
Turner, John B.,II, 99

U

U.S. Army, 9, 23, 40, 106
U.S. Coast Guard, 63
U.S. Congress, 31, 123
U.S. Merchant Marine Service, 84
U.S. Navy, 10, 61, 64, 65
U.S. Peace Corps, 75
U.S. Public Health Service, 73, 81, 91
U.S. Route 66, 69
Uniformed Services University of the Health Sciences, 10, 61
United Farm Workers, 87
University Hospital, 110, 117
University of Alaska Fairbanks, 43
University of Arkansas at Little Rock, 10
University of Arkansas for Medical Sciences Library, 32
University of Chicago, 85
University of Kentucky, 121
University of Miami, 121
University of Miami Medical School, 57
University of Michigan, 18, 31, 32
University of Minnesota, 37
University of Minnesota Hospital, 105
University of Minnesota Medical School, 73
University of Missouri, 107, 109, 110, 117
University of Missouri-Columbia, 10, 67, 81, 107, 110, 116

University of Missouri School of Journalism, 128
University of Texas at Austin, The, 44, 45, 46, 47, 48, 106
University of Utah Medical Center, 94, 97
University of Washington, 50, 123
Urban Horizons, 87
USS *Simon Lake*, 63
Utah, 9, 94, 95, 97, 98, 91, 119
Utah Capitol Building, 95
Utah Department of Health, 97

V

vaccination, 17
Vermont, 83, 101
Vesalius, Andreas, 17
Vienna, Austria, 19, 27
Vienna General Hospital, 19
Vietnam War, 33
Virchow, Rudolf, 19
Virgin Islands, 121
Virginia, 11, 57, 75
Virginia Polytechnic Institute, 57
Vogel, Christina Stanard, 128

W

Walls, Arch, 119
Walls, Jodie, 56
Walls, John, 56
Walls, Miranda, 56
Warren, John Collins, 19
Washington, 50, 63, 123
Washington, D.C., 25, 121, 122, 123
Washington University, 81, 116
Webster County Health Unit, 68
Webster County, Mo., 68, 103, 107
Welsch, Suzanne, 94
Wendover, Ky., 42
West Africa, 75
West, David M., 122
Westborne Mountain, 90
whooping cough, 63
Wichita, Kan., 11
Wilcox County, Ala., 9, 79, 83
Wilkinson, Nelda, Mrs., 4, 20
Will Mayfield College, 4
Willard, 119
Willard Committee, 34
Williamsburg, Ky., 89
Willingham, Mary, 80
Wisconsin, 21, 103, 107, 117, 122
Woman's Medical College of Pennsylvania, 30, 102
Wood, Grant, 99
World Conference on Tobacco and Health, 73
World Organization of Family Doctors, 123
World War I, 9, 40, 41
World War II, 29, 43, 67, 71, 106
World Wide Web, 7
Wyoming, 53

X

X-rays, 19

Y

Yale University, 13, 15, 27
Youmans, Gilbert, 117

Z

Zimble, James A., 64

About the Author

John R. Stanard
(Photo by Joe Craig)

*J*ohn R. Stanard's first books were *Butler County: A Pictorial History, Volumes I and II*, in 1993 and 1994. With his earlier background as a prize-winning reporter and photojournalist, the former editor and co-owner of his community's daily newspaper brings a special blend of skills to this latest project.

Stanard, a 1962 honored graduate of the University of Missouri School of Journalism, worked on the *Beaumont (Texas) Enterprise* and *The Minneapolis Star* before joining the staff of his family newspaper, the *Daily American Republic*, in Poplar Bluff, Mo. His parents and both of his grandfathers were newspaper writers and editors.

Since 1990, his editorial consulting assignments have included editing/writing seminars for press groups, publications judging, teaching classes on the print media for Linda Bloodworth-Thomason's Claudia Company, and editing Matt Chaney's heart-warming book, *My Name Is Mr. Ryan*, a historical account of the small Missouri town of Puxico and its state champion basketball teams.

Stanard and his wife, Vida, live in his hometown of Poplar Bluff. Their two children are Michael J. Stanard and Christina Stanard Vogel. When he's not writing, Stanard likes to fish and hunt the streams and hills of his beloved Missouri Ozarks.

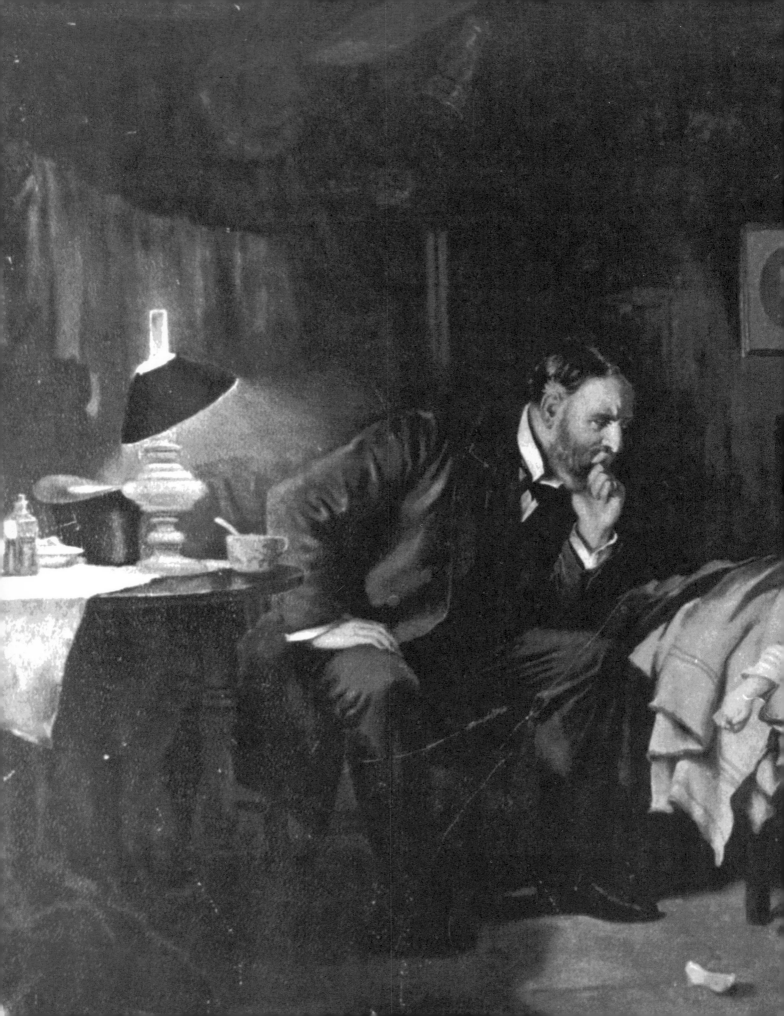